Schaum's Quick Guide to Great Presentations

Melody Templeton

Suzanne Sparks FitzGerald

McGraw-Hill

New York   San Francisco   Washington, D.C.   Auckland   Bogotá
Caracas   Lisbon   London   Madrid   Mexico City   Milan
Montreal   New Delhi   San Juan   Singapore
Sydney   Tokyo   Toronto

McGraw-Hill

A Division of The **McGraw·Hill** Companies

8 9 10 11 12 13 14 15 DOC/DOC 0 9 8 7 6 5

ISBN 0-07-022061-1

*The sponsoring editor for this book was Barbara Gilson, the editing supervisor was Fred
Dahl, the designer was Inkwell Publishing Services, and the production supervisor was
Pamela Pelton. It was set in Stone Serif by Inkwell Publishing Services.*

Printed and bound by R. R. Donnelley & Sons Company.

This book is printed on recycled, acid-free paper containing
a minimum of 50% recycled, de-inked fiber.

Contents

Schaum's Quick Guide
to Great Presentations

Part I

In the Beginning

Chapter I

Getting Started

As in any big project, often the hardest part of preparing your speech is getting started. It's best to start with the big picture in mind, and to do that you need to make some decisions.

Why Are You Speaking?

During the entire preparation process, keep the reason you're presenting in mind. To determine your purpose statement, consider these questions:

- What do you want your audience to know?
- What do you want your audience to feel?
- What do you want your audience to do?

Most reasons for speaking fall into 3 categories: to persuade, to inform (or teach), or to entertain. Most speaker's goals include a combination of these 3 reasons.

Now that you've determined your reasons, phrase them into a specific purpose statement. Here are some examples of a purpose statement:

I want my audience to understand the reasons for recycling newspapers and to take action by personally recycling!

I want my audience to understand the characteristics of 3 accounting methods.

I want my audience to believe that drug testing by employers is necessary in certain industries.

As you begin working on your presentation and decide what you want to accomplish, keep your purpose in mind. To help you stay focused, write out your purpose for speaking on every paper associated with your presentation—at the top of each page of your notes and on a sticky note on your computer screen. You'll have a goal, a focus, and a checkpoint.

Methods of Presenting

Now that you know why you're speaking, you must decide on the proper format.

Presentations come in many forms. You might speak in a rally to convince the listeners to vote for your candidate. You might conduct a session on "customer relations and dealing with difficult people" for a group of retailers. In a meeting, you might be asked, unexpectedly, to update your peers on the project you currently manage. You might even have to tell the crowds at a trade show about the advantages of the new "Slice and Dice" potato peeler! Different situations call for different formats. Let's look at 2 of the most common types.

Training Versus Public Speaking

The information in this book applies to trainers and public speaking students alike; however, there are some fundamental differences.

TRAINING

Definition

Training is a process, an intervention designed to change behavior. Effective training inside an organization takes place after a needs assessment. The purpose of a needs assessment is to determine specific problem areas in an organization and to address those problems.

Example

Human resource professionals gather data by interviewing the individuals or groups involved. Questionnaires or surveys may provide similar information. Sometimes the problem area is identified by observation alone. Based on the findings of the needs assessment, the human resource professional develops a training program.

Training programs are also given for the general public on topics of common interest like presentation skills, specific computer software packages or supervisory skills. Attendees can learn basic skills to transfer to their own specific situations.

Format

Training is interactive. The format of a training session usually includes a trainer introducing the program, going over the goals and objectives, and then using several methods of teaching the material before asking participants to practice what they've learned. Then the trainer gives participants feedback on their performance. The content usually includes several distinct sections, like Objectives, Materials, Time, and Methods. (The Exercises section at the end of each chapter is set up in a similar format.)

A training program may be ongoing, building on previously learned skills with each session. It may be a standalone program repeated for many different groups.

Time

Training may take place in an hour or less or take place in segments over weeks.

Materials

A trainer usually speaks from a training manual, which is similar to an actor's script in that the right side of the page contains the script and the left side lists the stage directions (what to do when saying these words).

Participants

Individuals or teams present training programs. They may be experts in the content that the session involves or experts in the process of training itself. The audience (usually a small group) can all be observed individually by the presenters. The presenters look for nonverbal reactions and may clarify information at any time during the presentation.

PUBLIC SPEAKING

Definition

Public speaking usually involves 1 person standing before an audience with the purpose of persuading, informing, or entertaining them.

Format

The simple format of a speech typically consists of an introduction, the body (which is separated into main and subpoints), and a conclusion. The speaker often speaks from notes carefully prepared from an outline. Sometimes, speakers use a manuscript to deliver their message. The presentation may be prepared well in advance and memorized, entirely off the cuff, or, most frequently extemporaneous. An *extemporaneous speech* is well prepared and follows a specific outline, but the words the speaker uses are chosen at the time of the presentation. It sounds natural.

Typically public speaking occurs in an isolated instance. Listeners hear your speech once, and if you give the same speech again, the audience is made up of individuals who are different from those in the first group.

Time

Public speaking is measured in minutes. Seldom does a speech go over 1 hour.

Materials

Speakers use notes to deliver speeches. The presenter may supplement materials with visual aids or hand-outs.

Participants

Normally only 1 person gives a speech. Panel presentations may include several people with one purpose who speak in sequence. The audience members may consist of only a handful or thousands.

Now that you know the basic differences between training and public speaking, you can easily adapt any information presented in this book. So let's get started.

An Easy Start

No method of preparing a presentation works every time. This simple technique seems to be almost universally successful with both students and other speakers in all fields. Even if you're a procrastinator, try this approach as soon *as you know you have to speak.*

Give yourself 10-15 minutes to focus on your topic. On a blank sheet of paper, write down as many things as you can think of that you might want to include in your presentation. Do not organize, eliminate, or think too hard on any item. Yes, we're talking about plain old brainstorming. Keep listing anything and everything you can possibly relate to your speech. As simple as it sounds, this 15-minute investment yields huge returns.

Once you have your brainstorming list, group the items into loose categories. Find items that seem to go together. If an item falls into more than 1 category, don't worry about it; you may mention this topic in entirely different ways in several categories. At this point, let natural groupings develop.

How It Works

Suppose you're speaking to a small group of employees who plan to take a business trip to Hong Kong. All the people in your group will take their families along and will combine a few days of business with a brief family vacation. Your responsibility is to tell them how to prepare for this trip. Your specific purpose might be:

> I will inform the audience of the necessary items to consider when preparing for an overseas family trip.

Your list of all the things you want to include might look like this:

Weather at time of trip

Passport or visa

Hotel reservations

Currency conversion rate

Family entertainment

Clothes—business and leisure

Allergy medicine for Sue

Pet to kennel

Stop mail

Travelers checks

Pay bills early

Suitcases for everyone

Pack

Transportation to and from airport

Ground transportation in Hong Kong

Learn language basics

List of emergency numbers

English-speaking guides

Walking shoes

Notify school of children's absence

Homework?

Flight length—snacks for children

Pack lap top

After reviewing your list, try to find natural groupings for your items. One group of categories might look like this:

Business

 Laptop

 Transportation—airport and in Hong Kong

 Business clothes

Family

 Passport

 Travel snacks for kids

 School notification

 Homework

 Walking shoes

Suitcases

Allergy medicine

Entertainment

Pack clothes

Hotel reservation

Home

Pet to kennel

House sitter

Pay bills

Stop mail

Emergency number lists

Some topics cross over both business and family categories:

Travelers checks

English travel guide

Learn language basics

After reviewing your lists, you may find a few items missing. Add them in! You may find that the family category is too long and might work better with 2 subcategories, such as "What to Plan For" and "Items to Take Along."

Go back now and check your specific purpose for speaking. If the groupings don't make sense for your purpose, eliminate those categories and choose new ones. Rearrange the points accordingly. Keep a note pad near you at all times to update your list as ideas occur to you.

Congratulations! Your speech preparation has begun painlessly. You have invested 15 minutes or so and you're off "square one"! If you have plenty of time before you give your presentation, here's some good news: You can put this brainstorming sheet away for a few days and not worry about it, but your subconscious will keep generating ideas! When you pull out your idea form again, you can usually pick up the preparation process right where you left off. Even if you change your format entirely, you have given yourself an excellent springboard.

Some of your anxiety should now disappear because you can see a light at the end of the tunnel! Try the following exercises to help you get started.

Exercises

PURPOSE STATEMENT

Objective

To learn to determine appropriate purpose statements for specific topics.

Method

Write your specific purpose in each situation.

1. You're speaking to junior high students about the hazards of smoking.

   _____

   _____

2. You're speaking to realtors on developing new sales markets.

   _____

   _____

3. You're speaking to engineers on how to give a speech.

   _____

   _____

4. You're speaking to engineers about the advantages of purchasing a new 3D drawing package.

   _____

   _____

5. You're speaking to college administrators about the dangers of hazing.

   _____

   _____

6. You're speaking to dining service employees on ways to generate creative problem-solving ideas.

   _____

   _____

7. You're speaking to neighborhood residents about the necessity for new high-power lines in their area.

_____

_____

8. You're speaking to dancers on the value of a good diet.

_____

_____

9. You're speaking to corporate executives about fund raising for a little boy from the community who was tragically burned in a house fire.

_____

_____

10. You're speaking to a singles group on the advantages of video dating.

_____

_____

PURPOSE STATEMENT

Objective

To gain skill in building a simple outline.

Method

On a blank sheet of paper, brainstorm an outline for the following topics:

1. Advantages of buying American cars.
2. Reasons to eat a healthy diet.
3. How to set up a new computer.

Allow just 15 minutes to generate ideas. When you have generated a list, find natural categories and from them determine and list your main points.

TRAINING OR PUBLIC SPEAKING?

Objective

To identify the appropriate time to use a training program or a speech.

Tools

No special tools are needed for this exercise.

Method

Read the following scenarios and determine, which calls for a training program, and which for a speech. Write either "Training" or "Public Speaking" in the spaces provided.

1. _____ A group of firefighters want to know how to improve their listening skills.

2. _____ A group of concerned parents want to know why their children are not receiving federally funded lunches.

3. _____ The American Kennel Club wants to know why you chose a Labrador retriever to be on the cover of the book you just published.

4. _____ You have been asked to help the engineers from a well known engineering company feel more comfortable giving project updates.

5. _____ The administrators from your college want to know why women choose your sorority over others on your campus.

6. _____ You have been selected to tell new employees how to fill out state and federal tax forms.

7. _____ You have been asked by a music professor to explain why Beethoven is a better composer than Yanni.

8. _____ You are newly elected to the board of trustees and have been asked to explain the goals of the board.

9. _____ One of the products your company produces has been fatal to 7 people. You must make this announcement to the public.

10. _____ A group of new realtors have asked you how a lock box works.

Answers are on the next page.

ANSWERS

1. Training
2. Public speaking
3. Public speaking
4. Training
5. Public speaking (A panel presentation would be a good choice since the experiences of a representative group could be given.)
6. Public speaking (This may be a surprising answer, but since filling out forms is a one-time-only experience for a new employee, the skills do not need to be well-learned. Employees can simply follow the instructions in a clearly presented informative speech that is supplemented with visual aids as examples. They can then easily accomplish the task.)
7. Public speaking
8. Public speaking
9. Public speaking (This situation requires an extremely carefully crafted statement that minimizes the damage to the image of your company, while maximizing the company's concern for the situation. This statement would most likely be read to the media and public at large. A question-and-answer period would follow, in which questions would be answered with care.)
10. Training (This could be a very brief training session including a hands-on demonstration.)

Chapter 2

Fear Fighting

When most people find out they have to give a presentation, they usually do 1 of 3 things: Try to get out of it, procrastinate, or start working on it. Usually, they choose option 3 only after they fail at the first 2.

Fear is the primary motivator for the first 2 responses. Usually we fear things that we're unfamiliar with. Since we spend so much of our time talking, why does the thought of speaking in public fill us with dread?

Sources of Fear

- *Looking foolish:* Often, we simply fear we'll do something that will make us look ridiculous. We might forget what to say, mispronounce words, break into a cold sweat, or trip on the way to the podium.

- *Being stared at:* Walking to the front of the room and looking at all the eyes looking back can be very intimidating. Being the center of attention brings out the natural shyness of many inexperienced speakers.

- *Fear of the unknown:* A new situation can cause anxiety. Having an audience watch as you navigate through new territory can be a major obstacle for inexperienced speakers.

- *Negative past experiences:* If we've been embarrassed on stage even once, that memory is burned into our brains. A humiliating experience as far back as grade school can live on forever.

A Quick Quiz

You may fear aspects of presenting. An impending presentation may be exciting, but it may also bring on feelings of dread. Here is a short quiz to determine what gives you the anxiety.

Rate yourself according to the following scale:

1–strongly disagree   2–disagree   3–neutral
4–agree   5–strongly agree

1. _____ The night before a presentation, I cannot sleep.

2. _____ I frequently contribute to discussions at work or in class.

3. _____ I like to help others learn things by teaching or instructing them.

4. _____ I avoid situations in which I might have to give an impromptu speech.

5. _____ When talking to people, I find it hard to look people in the eye.

6. _____ I get very uncomfortable when I'm in a situation that involves a heated debate and I might have to get involved.

7. _____ Others have made positive comments about my speaking ability.

8. _____ I have had at least one very embarrassing experience when speaking.

9. _____ I am intimidated in a job interview.

10. _____ Asking someone I admire to discuss a topic that interests me is fun.

11. _____ I can only speak from a written manuscript.

12. _____ I'm comfortable when I'm acting.

13. _____ I'd like to do stand-up comedy.

14. _____ I'm comfortable selling things to others.

15. _____ I'd rather go to the dentist, pay taxes, and clean closets than give a presentation!

As you review the way you rated yourself, try to determine how much anxiety you have about speaking. Look at the way you rated these questions between 1 and 5 to determine just how strongly you feel about each question.

- Is your fear related to specific situations like impromptu speaking, or is it present for all presentations? (Questions 1, 2, and 4)
- Do the size and nature of who is in the audience affect your fear? (Questions 3 and 10)
- Does the persuasive nature of an interview or debate scare you most? (Questions 6, 9, and 14)
- Do you telegraph your anxiety? (Question 5 and 7)
- Do you have residual fear from an event in your past? (Question 8)
- Do you feel more comfortable if you know each line you'll say in advance? Are you more comfortable if you assume the character of someone else? (Questions 11 and 12)
- Is simple survival your primary motive? (Question 15)

Try to find a pattern to your answers to decide if you should focus on specific speaking situations. The more precisely you can identify your most anxiety-producing situations, the more success you will have in finding methods to deal with them.

Methods to Combat Fear

Research shows that speaking before a group is consistently listed as number one on the list of things that people say cause them fear. Public speaking is more frightening than heights, insects, divorce, financial problems, and even death!

So how can you deal with anxiety? Consider the Olympic athlete who knows she must compete before thousands of spectators and millions more on television. She may feel pressure to perform, which could turn into fear or failure. To perform at her best, she trains carefully and extensively.

To combat presentation jitters, think of yourself as an Olympic speaker in training. Choose workout options that you think will help you.

PREPARATION

An Olympic athlete can't start preparing for competition a few days before the event. Neither can a good speaker. Begin gathering information as soon as you know your presentation date. Even though you don't have to start preparing your speech immediately, keeping a list of ideas that you generated in Chapter 1 will help the project come together. Get some ideas into the back of your mind as soon as possible.

PRACTICE

Many inexperienced speakers actually skip this step because practicing itself can be frightening. Going over the presentation in your head does not count as a *real* practice session. You'll need to stand up, look out at an imaginary audience, and project loudly. Repeat each movement and use your notes exactly as you will during your real presentation.

Perhaps the most important practice tip is to stand before a video camera to practice. You can review your "game tapes" to get an "audience's eye view" of how you actually perform. A coach can repeatedly tell you about distracting habits you may have, but the critique doesn't become real until you see it for yourself.

Video cameras are usually easy to find. If you are going to speak in a classroom, it may be equipped with a camera. If you're speaking in a business situation, most companies have a camera you can borrow. Public or college libraries often have cameras that you can use in the library for practice. If all else fails, most of us know a relative or neighbor who takes those annoying videos at every party or gathering. You might borrow the camera and tripod from one of them.

Some of us resist videotaping because we're afraid to see what we really look like. Think of it this way: Wouldn't you rather see those little annoying habits now, in private, and correct them before you stand before your peers, your manager, or other executives? You can correct the great majority of bad habits fairly easily.

FAMILIARITY

Do you remember your first day of school or work? Everything was new and probably a little scary. Within a few days, even if you didn't like the teacher or the job, at least you knew what to expect. The anxiety associated with the "newness" disappeared. Simply being in an environment for a while makes us more comfortable.

The same philosophy applies to performing. The Olympic athlete competes many times before the big event, having trained repeatedly in a place very similar to the setting where she'll actually compete. She has been on a court, rink, slope, or track enough that she knows what to expect, so that many aspects of competing seem routine and comfortable. A speaker must practice in a room similar to the room in which she'll actually speak. Whether your speech will be held in a classroom, conference room, or auditorium, practice in a room that most nearly duplicates the real situation. This reduces your anxiety. Do this several times until you become familiar and comfortable with the environment.

REFRAMING

To gain some control of your anxiety, change how you define your feelings. Instead of defining your anxiety as fear, try calling it excitement. Imagine the Olympian stepping up to perform. She needs a degree of excitement and adrenaline for a great performance. No excitement might appear as no enthusiasm for the performance. No one wants to watch an unenthusiastic performance.

Reframe the image of giving the presentation from something you *have to do* to a picture of something you *get to do*. Just viewing the speech as an opportunity, not a threat, makes the process easier.

VISUALIZATION

Close your eyes and "see" yourself standing before your audience. See yourself looking confident, competent, and credible. See the audience smiling and nodding as they comprehend your point. Feel yourself enjoying the experience. Mentally go through every step of the presentation from stepping up before the group to hearing the applause of the appreciative audience. Imagine yourself walking back to your seat with a satisfied smile on your face, and feel the joy of having done an excellent presentation. *See* success!

DIET

Believe it or not, what you eat before you speak can affect your presentation. Consider eating a light meal before the performance. An empty stomach does not react well to anxiety. A heavy meal might make you sluggish and make your stomach churn as you start to speak. A light meal that is high in protein or carbohydrates usually gets you off to a good start.

Even if you love coffee, don't consume too much caffeine. Your natural adrenaline provides as much of a "jump start" as you need. Too much caffeine causes jitters and makes your hands and knees shake. Beware of eating sugar or drinking sugar-loaded beverages before you speak. Sugar coats the throat and may make speaking without clearing your throat difficult. Beware of similar problems after consuming milk products.

EXERCISE

If you anticipate that your hands or knees will start to shake during the presentation, consider isometric exercises. As you wait to stand up to give your presentation, make tight fists, hold them for a count of five and release. Repeat several times. If possible, walk around a little before you begin your presentation. Pacing in a private area can help get rid of excess adrenaline. Take deep breaths through your nose and exhale slowly through your mouth. Do *not* hyperventilate; just breathe deeply enough to relax.

ACCEPTANCE

Keep in mind that some degree of anxiety is actually necessary to give a good presentation. The adrenaline you bring to the podium can be converted from anxiety to energy. A speaker without energy and enthusiasm has little chance of keeping the interest of the audience. So welcome your butterflies!

Keep in mind that everyone who speaks feels some anxiety. It's something we *want* to have and can learn to appreciate. The famous writer William Jennings Bryan put it this way: "Should the time ever come when I walk out before an audience without feeling any stage fright, I would then know I had lost the essential qualification for speaking."

The best way to combat fear of speaking is to *do* it. Create as many opportunities to speak as you can. Often civic groups, the PTA, and volunteer organizations look for speakers. Even participating in classes and meetings at work provides an opportunity to speak. The experience gets more comfortable every time.

The process of being an Olympic speaker "in training" can convert the fear you may feel into positive energy. Use that positive energy to make your best appearance yet! Go for your own gold!

The following exercises help you fight the fear and go for *your* gold!

Exercises

A LOOK AT YOUR PAST

Objective

To apply coping skills learned in the past to the current speaking situation.

Method

Relax and get into a comfortable position. Prepare to sit alone with your thoughts for about 15 minutes. Think of times in your life when you were willing to invest time and effort improving a skill you needed and/or enjoyed. You may have wanted to improve your ability in sports, music, computing, art, etc. Think of a time when you were very anxious about something you now do well. Ask yourself these questions:

- Can you describe the situation?

  _____

  _____

- How did you handle your anxiety at first?

  _____

  _____

- What helped the most?

  _____

  _____

- What techniques didn't work?

  _____

  _____

- Why is it easier for you now?

  _____

  _____

- How can you apply the same techniques to speaking?

  _____

  _____

Example

- Can you describe the situation

  I was afraid to kayak. I fell out of a canoe once and was not hurt, but I swallowed some water and felt humiliated in front of friends. Being in any kind of boat on the water became scary to me.

- How did you handle your anxiety at first?

  At first I simply avoided kayaking even though my friends went often and enjoyed themselves. I watched them from the shore and felt stupid for not being able to join them.

- What helped the most?

  My friend Steve finally convinced me to try going on the water once. He helped me strap on a life vest and showed me boating safety techniques. We went out in the kayak on a day when no one was around, so that no one would laugh.

- What techniques didn't work?

  Two of my friends made fun of me for being such a chicken. That just made it worse.

- Why is it easier for you now?

  Once we got on to the water, I realized just how stable some kayaks are. I thought all of them were white water kayaks. I had seen them on TV and thought I had to roll over if I went out in one. Now I realize how irrational this belief was since none of my friends ever rolled while I was watching them. Since I took the risk that first time I found out kayaking is safe and fun. I also realized that I am in control in my own boat.

- How can you apply the same techniques to speaking?

  Sometimes you just have to do something to understand what it's like. I have to give a speech for my sorority next week and I'm going to call Steve to help me again. I can practice with him in private and get his feedback. He's kind and supportive and that might make me feel like I have a "speech life vest" so I can't sink while I'm speaking! I really want to be an officer next year, and I'll have to speak often to get nominated and even more after I'm elected. If I can get comfortable with speaking, maybe I'll feel in control when I'm with an audience—like I feel in control in my kayak!

SELF-FULFILLING PROPHECY

Objectives

To identify specific fears associated with speaking.

To plan personal strategies for dealing with anxiety.

Method

We typically get what we expect in this life. It's called self-fulfilling prophecy. When we get a picture of ourselves clearly placed in our mind's eye, we then act accordingly to make that picture come true. For instance, students who are told that they are stupid often believe they are stupid. They then start to believe that they can't learn and have a corresponding drop in grades. When students with the same IQ scores are told that they are very bright, they act accordingly and begin to achieve better grades.

Complete the following questions. Be as specific and detailed as possible to get a complete picture of exactly what you fear and how to address those fears.

The worst things that could happen to me when giving my speech are:

1. _____
2. _____
3. _____
4. _____
5. _____
6. _____
7. _____
8. _____

If these things were to happen, how would I feel? (Be specific about exactly what you fear. If you can identify your specific fears, you can get at the root cause.)

1. _____
2. _____
3. _____
4. _____
5. _____
6. _____
7. _____
8. _____

What specific steps can I take to address these fears? Be exact and detailed about what you can do to keep your negative concerns from happening.

1. _____
2. _____
3. _____
4. _____

5. _____
6. _____
7. _____
8. _____

If I apply each of those techniques, what will happen and how will I feel? (Focus on your exact positive feelings.)

1. _____
2. _____
3. _____
4. _____
5. _____
6. _____
7. _____
8. _____

Go back to the list of the worst things that could happen to you. Imagine each one of them happening and blow them up to extreme proportions in your mind. See them getting worse and worse until the whole picture is so absurd that you have to laugh at yourself.

1. _____
2. _____
3. _____
4. _____
5. _____
6. _____
7. _____
8. _____

If you have strong fears about presenting, doing this exercise is important—actually writing out each step. Once you realize what the fear is really about and that typically we blow our fears out of proportion, the situation becomes more manageable.

VISUALIZATION

Objectives

To learn the feelings associated with a positive speaking experience.

To see yourself as comfortable standing before an audience.

Method

Read this exercise completely and be very familiar with it before you begin. Get comfortable and relaxed in a quiet place. You may sit or lie down. You may choose to have quiet music in the background (instrumental only).

Close your eyes and see yourself on the day of your presentation. You look relaxed and peaceful. You're wearing clean, neat, attractive clothes. Your shoes are polished and comfortable and your hair is neat and attractive. You know you look great!

See yourself walking into the room where you're speaking. The audience is smiling and applauding. They are eager to hear what you have to say. As you walk to the front of the room, you feel confident and enthusiastic. As you turn to face the group, you take a deep breath, exhale, and begin your introduction. The audience is listening attentively and looking at you with friendly eyes.

As you move through the main points of your presentation, your confidence soars. You know your voice is strong, your gestures are comfortable, and the audience is nodding in agreement. Standing in front of the audience feels comfortable. *You* are the person the audience wants to hear. As the speech comes to a close, the audience applauds for you. As you listen to the applause, you know you were successful. You were confident, knowledgeable, and professional. You feel a rush of adrenaline—just as though you have won the gold medal!

Slowly open your eyes and quietly let yourself feel the joy of a successful experience!

CHANGING EXPECTATIONS

Objectives

To understand that your expectations affect your experience.

To see yourself as comfortable standing before an audience.

Method

Preferably, you have been sitting in the same room for several minutes as you try this exercise.

Look around you and try to find 5 blue things. Make sure you get 5. Now look again and find 5 more blue things. Now that you have 10 things on your mental list, ask yourself this question: Did I see anything that I hadn't noticed before the exercise?

Most likely, you saw something that was there all along. You simply had not really "seen" it before you looked for it. If you were looking for yellow things, you would have found yellow things. The point of this exercise is to make real to you the philosophy that we find exactly what we look for! If you expect to be anxious, you probably will be anxious. If you expect to be relaxed, you will find that you are relaxed. If you are scared that you will blank out and keep thinking about blanking out, chances are good that somewhere in your presentation, you'll forget what to say. Don't think in terms of "I won't blank out." Think of "I'll remember all that I need to know." Never phrase your affirmations in the negative.

From now on, choose to think positively. Look for the positive things and you'll find them. Choose to focus on the good things that can come from speaking. Think of yourself as confident and competent! Here's the key: You don't have to really believe these positive things—just pretend to believe them. Believing *will* work.

Chapter 3

Getting Acquainted with Your Audience

Developing your presentation with the audience in mind is probably the most critical step in inventing your speech. Your presentation is given for your audience, not you. The audience primarily determines your success. No matter how much you know about a topic, how enthusiastic you are, or what importance you place on what you have to say, if an audience doesn't think your presentation is good, they're right. It isn't good—for that audience.

A speech designed to convince an audience to attend a Phish concert might get a very positive response from a group of college students, but would probably be inappropriate for an audience of World War II veterans. A message that might compel a structural engineer might bore a pharmacist or a dancer. The more you know about the group who will listen to you, the greater your chances of success.

A good audience analysis is the core of your preparation. The language you use, the examples you choose, and the general presentation style you adopt should be influenced by the nature of the audience. Some things you'll want to know about the audience include the demographics or vital statistics, the attitudes, values and interests, and the situation that brings them together.

Demographics

AGE

You'll want to know the age range of your audience so that you can determine some of their shared life experiences.

Example

An audience who was in the United States in the late 1960s does not need as much background on the topic of the Watergate affair as an audience born after 1970. Language patterns and appropriate examples vary with the age group you address.

GENDER

Is your audience predominately one gender or evenly mixed? Choose examples and language appropriate for everyone.

Example

For a mixed gender audience, you do not want to use an example of getting a nail wrap.

If you choose an example that is specific to one gender, try to follow it with another more general example or one specific to the other gender.

EDUCATION LEVEL

The audience's level of education should influence your language choices.

Examples

An audience with college or postgraduate education might be more responsive to complex reasoning and to cultural or literary references than a high-school-educated audience.

Concrete language is more effective with audiences with lower educational levels.

Do not talk down to your audience under any circumstances. Simply choose appropriate words.

POLITICAL AFFILIATION AND RELIGION

How liberal or conservative the audience is can help you make predictions about how to appeal to them. Topics relating to religion and politics are usually emotionally charged for most people. Be careful not to negatively arouse your audience with a comment you haven't thought through.

Example

A Catholic, Republican audience will probably oppose the easy availability of abortions. A group with different religious affiliations will likely be more open to that subject.

OCCUPATION

Try to use examples to which the audience can relate.

Example

Use sales examples for retailers and medical examples for doctors.

INCOME LEVEL

Knowing the average income level can help you adapt a message with a financial focus. It also can help you avoid embarrassing or insulting the audience.

Examples

Appealing to a lower-income audience to invest in an expensive IRA or contribute thousands of dollars to a political campaign is far more challenging than addressing the same topics to a middle- or upper-income audience.

Low- to moderate-income audiences are frequently more responsive to contributing to grassroots or social causes than wealthy audiences.

ETHNICITY

Your choice of language may be appropriate for one ethnic group and not another. Some cultures expect more politeness and respect than others. Some cultures expect a speaker to talk and dress formally while others feel comfortable with a casual approach. If you simply use basic human respect for everyone, you can eliminate many potential problems or misunderstandings.

GEOGRAPHIC LOCATION

Match your message to the locale.

Examples

Use an example of eating grits and cornbread in Marion, South Carolina and an example of raising cattle in Colorado or Texas.

Don't try to convince people in Florida to buy snow tires.

Don't expect an audience in Arizona to buy a lot of umbrellas.

Caution! Only assume so much. Because you're speaking to a group of women, do not assume they're all mothers or find children's issues interesting. If you're speaking to 65-year-olds, don't assume they are retired and free to travel. Assuming too much is a primary cause of "foot in mouth disease."

Attitudes, Values and Interests

Determine as much as you can about the following things to make your message as effective as possible.

KNOWLEDGE

- Will your audience understand your message?
- Is their knowledge technical or general?
- Do they share a common knowledge base, or do some know more than others?

Determine what they share in common. It's a good idea to start talking at a level they all understand and quickly bring the less knowledgeable members up to the basic level needed to make your points.

INTEREST

- Why are they here?
- Is it because they choose to attend or because they are required to attend?
- Do they want you to succeed?
- Are they friendly or hostile?

An audience who wants to be there is already motivated to listen. Those who would rather be anywhere else need to be encouraged to listen. They want to know, "What's in it for them?" Answer that question as early as possible. Hostile audiences should feel that you understand their position even though it may differ from yours.

LANGUAGE

- Do you share the same language base with the audience members?
- Do they know acronyms?
- Are they from another state or country?

Make sure you aren't using terminology they don't understand. Early in your presentation, define terms and acronyms that some in the audience might not comprehend.

INFLUENCE

- Who in the group is the decision maker?
- Who is an informal leader?
- Is your message threatening to the decision maker?

Make sure you know the key players. Gear the message to the most powerful members of the audience.

Hint: Those who hold the highest title are not always the most powerful. Make sure everyone saves face and the outcome can be viewed as a win–win.

RELATIONSHIP

- Do the group members know each other?
- What is their history with each other? With you?
- Is there tension in the group?

A group that meets regularly for social reasons usually wants a speaker to deliver a short, interesting, entertaining message. Highly social groups have been known to start socializing during the presentation if it lasts longer than anticipated! If the speaker is well known to the audience, a personal approach is very effective. The exception to this occurs when the message is negative. Bad news requires a formal presentation style.

CONCERNS

- Why do the members of the audience *want* to know about your topic?

- What do they *need* to know?
- Why they should listen to you?
- Do they see you as credible?

Always tell the audience what it needs to know. Sometimes, that message needs to be wrapped in a coating of what it wants to know. (This is a good idea only as long as what the audience wants to know is true, ethical, and can be used to support your point.)

Example

On the first beautiful day of spring, an audience of college juniors may *want* to hear that class is canceled for the day. What it *needs* to hear may be the planned lecture because the material is on the upcoming test!

The audience must see you as credible. You can earn that label based on education, reputation, and knowledge. If you have no credibility with a particular audience, someone else should present for you. Good ethics are essential for long-lasting credibility.

Situation

WHY THEY ARE GATHERED

Example

Is this group meeting because they all oppose a new mobile phone tower scheduled to be erected on a neighboring property? Is it your job to represent the phone company and convince them that this tower will benefit them? If so, you will most likely have a hostile audience.

On the other hand, if the group members have met regularly for some time and primarily socialize at each event, they will probably be receptive to listening to a short presentation. They may even expect to be entertained before returning to the social portion of the gathering.

EXPECTATIONS

- Do they want to be entertained?
- Do they expect you to be formal or casual?

- Are they expecting a "sales pitch"?
- Do they prefer their presentations to be given in a Q-and-A format?

ULTERIOR MOTIVES

- Were you asked to speak for a reason unknown by you?

Examples

If you are a car dealer, do they hope to get deep discounts?

Were you asked to speak as a favor to your "Uncle Bob" because he's a big contributor to the organization and the group just wants to "butter up" Uncle Bob?

THEIR GROUP HISTORY

- Do they know each other well?
- Do they like each other?
- Does anyone have a political agenda?

Group members who do not know each other act more formally than a group already on friendly terms. If they don't know each other, they attempt to learn each other's position on the topic. A friendly group is more casual and the group as a whole probably vocalizes more than strangers.

CONTEXT

- What is the environment? Consider the politics, the turf, the day of the week, the time of day, etc.
- Are they hungry and anxious for lunch?
- Are they full and sleepy from a big meal and sitting in a warm room?

Adapt the design of your presentation to the setting.

Examples

Do not schedule a long-winded speaker or a lecture-style presentation immediately after lunch.

If you want a commitment to a decision, you're likely to get it more quickly when the group is hungry and ready to break for lunch.

Speedy decisions also happen on a Friday afternoon.

Notes:
- Do not expect an audience to give you its full attention at such times.
- If 2 people in the room hold long-standing, opposing political issues, do not seat them next to each other or directly across a table from each other.

SIZE OF THE GROUP

The larger your audience, the more formal your presentation should be. Prepare to use formal language and formal body language in a large group. A large audience usually requires that the speaker stand rather than sit and lecture rather than hold a discussion.

Note: You need to know the head count to distribute handouts.

Gathering Audience Information

Now that you've discovered what you need to learn about the audience, you have to obtain that information. There are many resources available, and the more of them you can use, the more accurate your information is likely to be. Try to learn about your audience from these sources:

YOUR OWN HISTORY WITH THE GROUP

This is effective for any ongoing group, such as a class, work unit, club, or organization. Keep your eyes and ears open for information. Why are you involved with this group? What common bond brings this group of people together?

THE PERSON WHO ASKED YOU TO SPEAK

Usually this person is a member of the group or at least knows the people involved. Ask pointed questions about the audience. Try to determine if there are any hidden reasons for asking you to speak. Sometimes groups just need to have an "entertainment portion of the meeting," and they would prefer a light, noncontroversial topic rather than a passionate persuasive speech.

OTHER SPEAKERS WHO HAVE PREVIOUSLY ADDRESSED THIS GROUP

Other speakers might be able to tell you if the group is friendly or hostile, formal or informal, involved in your topic or disinterested. Other speakers can help in telling you about the acoustics of the room.

WRITTEN MATERIAL ABOUT THE GROUP

This may be the least effective of the methods listed because the communication is one-way (you cannot ask questions) and the information may be out of date. If you search carefully and double check your information, you may, however, discover valuable information in print.

GRAPEVINE INFORMATION

Don't totally trust this source. Carefully check out anything you hear, including rumors, second-hand stories, and assumptions. If the information is accurate, you may have discovered a gold mine. If it is inaccurate, you could embarrass yourself. Newspapers and television stations have had to publicly retract stories that proved untrue. Reputations have been damaged and jobs have been lost. Find 2 reliable sources—at least 1 in writing—before including information you're not positive is true.

Once you have learned as much as you can about your audience, you can begin to use this information in preparing your speech.

The following exercises will help you learn ways to get acquainted with your audience.

Exercises

DEMOGRAPHICS

Objectives

To determine demographic data about your audience.

To interpret what this data means to your presentation.

Method

Using the methods listed in the chapter (interviews, observations, and questionnaires), record your answers to the following questions regarding your audience:

1. What is the average age and age range?
2. What is the average education level?
3. What is the gender ratio?
4. What is the ethnic diversity?
5. What cultural differences are represented?
6. What is the dominant socioeconomic class?
7. What religions are represented?
8. Where are they from geographically?
9. Why are they meeting?
10. How many are in the group?
11. Have you had prior contact with this audience?

INTERPRETATION

Based on the information you have gathered, determine the answers to the following questions:

1. What is the audiences interest in your topic?
2. Will its attitude toward your message be positive, negative, or neutral?
3. What is its level of understanding of your topic?
4. What do audience members expect from your presentation?
5. What is their attitude toward you as a speaker?

ADAPTING YOUR PRESENTATION

Objective

To apply the audience's demographic information to preparing your presentation.

Method

Based on the information you know about your audience, write your answers to the following questions. Keep your specific topic and goal in mind for each question.

1. What kind of introduction will get its attention?
   _____

2. What examples will this group respond to? _____
   _____

3. How will you develop your main points for this audience?
   _____

   _____

4. How will you adapt your delivery for this group—language, pace, volume, etc.? _____
   _____

5. How should you dress for your presentation?_____
   _____

THE TARGET AUDIENCE

Objective

To show examples of adapting a message to specific audiences.

Method

1. Advertisers spend much of their time and money studying which messages appeal to certain audiences. Go to the library to review the magazine section. Choose five or six magazines that appear to target audiences of different interests and demographics.

   Example
   Choose magazines on upscale travel, sports, finance, teen fashion, spirituality, and healthy lifestyle.

   Try to determine the target audiences based on the visuals chosen to represent the products as well as the text and word choices used in the ads.

2. If possible, find an ad for the same product in two very different publications. How do the ads vary? Chances are the audience can't relate to the ad prepared for someone else.

Example

Why might the ad in the finance magazine not persuade the readers of a teen fashion magazine to buy the product?

3. Choose another product and jot down ways you might design an ad to appeal to different audiences.

Example

A multiple vitamin might be represented as a part of a body-building program that features a picture of an athlete with well-defined muscles and an excellent physique in a sports magazine. The same multiple vitamin might be pictured in a convenient, small container for the health-conscience traveler.

As you observe the different ways advertisers appeal to audiences of different demographics and interests, you will become more aware of techniques you can use to adjust your style in delivering any message.

Chapter 4

Gathering Data

Linda stood before an audience looking professional and sounding confident and convincing. Still, for some reason, the audience seemed restless and disinterested.

Having no idea what was making them uncomfortable, she hurried to reach her conclusion and ended her speech. A few members of the audience left grumbling and one of her listeners came up to the podium to ask a question. As soon as Linda answered the question, she realized, to her embarrassment, what had happened.

Linda made the humiliating error of quoting inaccurate information. A coworker had given her data that Linda didn't check. All it was missing was a zero, but that little zero made a huge difference in her findings.

The data used to support ideas is critical to your success. Its accuracy, the credibility of your source, its relevance, and how you present the data all contribute to your credibility. Never forget your ethical obligation to yourself and the audience to be accurate and fair in your presentation.

How to Choose Data

The amount of information available today is overwhelming. How do you choose what to use? You cannot include something just because it is interesting. When you find something you're not sure you want to mention, ask yourself:

- How does this support my purpose statement?

- How does this relate to my point?
- Will including this material help lead logically to my conclusion?

   Two hints help you begin to gather information from various sources:

1. Start with the most current sources and work back in time. This shows you the current thinking on the ideas you're researching and prevents you from pursuing dead ends.
2. Research general information on your topic and work to the specific. The general information gives you good background to prepare your specific points.

Sources of Data

You can find data in many sources, including:

- The library.
- The Internet.
- Printed information provided by organizations.
- Interviews.
- Your own experience.

LIBRARY AND INTERNET

   When you visit the library, your best resource is the research librarian. Librarians don't know the answer to every question (although sometimes they seem to!). They do, however, know how to help you find almost any answer. They can help you overcome many fears you have about finding information. Nearly every library has computerized catalogs for books and periodicals. Most libraries also have pamphlets on how to access the resources available to you. In the library, you can find encyclopedias, *The Guiness Book of World Records*, books of quotations, books specifically written as resources for speakers, newspapers from around the world, and many other sources of information. Go in, look around, and ask questions. Make your trip to the library an adventure. Remember one thing: Do not expect the librarian to do your work for you!

The Internet is like a huge library, full of more information than you ever thought existed. You can access international newspapers, see what's happening at NASA, and talk to your friend in Peoria by e-mail. If you would like a recipe from Martha Stewart or investment advice from Dean Witter-Morgan Stanley, you can just pull it up on your screen. The Internet, however, doesn't have a central information center like a librarian, nor does it have any "quality control." Anything can be printed on the Internet, regardless of accuracy or good taste. Be careful of the information you find here.

Finding information on the Internet can begin with visiting a search engine, which sorts information by the key words you request. Search engines come and go and are sometimes as dynamic as the Internet itself. Here are some of the most popular ones:

- Yahoo (http://www.yahoo.com)
- Alta Vista (http://www.altavista.digital.com)
- Excite NetSearch (http//www.excite.com)
- Lycos (http//www.lycos.com)
- metacrawler (http//www.metacrawler.com)

Each of these search engines has instructions for the best way to find information. Not all search engines function the same way; so check the specific instructions for each one until you're comfortable using it. Publications with lists of Web sites are released constantly. (And they quickly become outdated.) If you'll frequently be working on the Internet, you may want to purchase a current edition. Be sure to check the copyright date.

ORGANIZATIONAL MATERIALS

Materials provided by organizations may include annual reports, marketing materials, and internal communication. You can write or call, asking to have information sent, or you might ask someone who works for a company to share information. Do not ask for confidential information!

Remember that materials published by an organization will portray a positive image of that organization.

INTERVIEWS

Informational interviewing is an excellent way to get first-hand information, Some hazards are associated with interviews: The person may not tell you the truth or might not show up. Or you may think the information they tell you is generalizable to a larger population when, in reality, it is simply the opinion of one person. As long as you keep these things in mind, interviewing can be fun and very rewarding.

If you are a college student, you will find that in general people are more willing to talk with you now than at any other time in your life—unless you become rich and famous! In the last few years, public speaking students at Villanova University have been given an assignment to interview someone they find interesting. They have talked with such well-known people as Alan Bean, Nancy Reagan, Kathie Lee Gifford, Newt Gingrich, Chris Berman, William Casey, the musical group Phish, Whitey Ford, and many, many other people who were gracious enough to share their time with a college student.

If you choose to interview someone, follow these simple rules:

- Start scheduling *early*. People are busy and most of them schedule everything well in advance. Don't expect to be the interviewee's main priority.

- Be clear about your purpose for the interview.

- Prepare your questions in advance. Know what you want to ask and how you will phrase your questions. At the same time, allow for plenty of flexibility in your interview. What the person wants to tell you may be much more interesting than what you thought you would discuss!

- Take no more than 15 minutes for your interview and tell the person that is all you expect from them when you call for your appointment.

- Dress appropriately for the interview and honor the individual's time.

- Most people don't like to be taped. Try to record the essence of your conversation in notes *immediately* after the interview. If you choose to tape, ask permission first.

- Send a thank-you note after the interview. Many people forget this courtesy. Make yourself stand out by remembering.

PERSONAL EXPERIENCE

The power of a personal experience is very strong. Think of your reaction to Christopher Reeves speaking about improvements in our ability to treat spinal cord injuries. Sarah Brady commands credibility when she speaks about gun control issues. Sometimes, the most effective speakers on the topics of drug, alcohol, or food addiction are former addicts. The personal experience of someone who has faced the issues you're discussing can serve as excellent information to add to your presentation.

Caution: Be careful not to get caught up in the "drama" of the story. You can spend too much time and give too many details when the situation is very close to your own life.

Types of Data

EXAMPLES, STORIES, AND QUOTES

Use an example or story to explain or clarify a point. An example is *not proof* of something. The story you tell should be relevant and should simply underscore your point. Examples and stories add "human interest" to your presentation. Effective stories are usually either poignant, tender, or funny. The many sources of stories range from real life experiences, through magazines, to books of stories complied for speakers. Sometimes the best materials come from obscure sources. Don't rule out anything (in good taste) until you've looked it over.

Birds and Blooms magazine recently published a letter from a reader who told the story of a woman who prepared

red-colored sugar water to feed her hummingbirds. She stored the sugar water in the refrigerator until one day her husband complained that the Kool Aid sure didn't have much flavor! This story could be used to illustrate communication issues in the household or to introduce a presentation on the country's most popular hobby—bird watching.

Quotes also add human interest and drama to your presentation. Quoting someone well-known or considered a credible source can give you credibility. Quoting someone who is not well respected or whose character is questionable is not a good idea. In some cases, the source of your quote may not be well-known, but the content supports your message. If you have no reason to doubt the character of the source, you can use the quote; just choose unknown sources carefully. Ironically, the person most often quoted in speeches seems to be the one known as Anonymous.

STATISTICS

It seems that there's a statistic for everything. If you've ever watched a television broadcast of a sport that you don't know much about, you may have heard the announcers listing a string of numbers that made no sense to you. The sports industry and the government may use more statistics than any other group in existence. (There's probably a statistic on this somewhere!)

But just what are statistics? *Statistics* are numerical data compiled in a way that makes the data meaningful. Effective use of statistics can clarify, support, and add powerful impact to your points. Improper use can make your presentation boring and unbelievable. Most of us know that statistics can be construed to "prove" almost any point, valid or not!

Example

Did you know that you can prove that white bread is the healthiest kind of bread because it is fortified with more vitamins and minerals than any other kind? Did you also know that you can prove that whole wheat bread is the healthiest kind of bread because it's highest in fiber and has fewer additives?

Be careful of how you use statistics and data. Make sure to cite the source of any statistics you mention in your presentation.

FACTS

Facts are also an important source of data. A *fact* is something that is true and can be proven.

Example

Fact: The white house is located at 1600 Pennsylvania Avenue.

Fact: The capitol of Alaska is Juneau

Fact: Margaret Thatcher was Prime Minister of Great Britain from 1979 to 1990.

Obviously you need to present accurate facts. If they aren't, you will have no credibility with your audience.

Double check all the information you gather for your presentation. With good, reliable, information you're well on your way to a successful presentation.

Try the following exercises to help you get started.

Exercises

FINDING SOURCES

Objective

To become successful and comfortable finding good resources of information.

Method

This exercise has no right answers (except number 8, which has more than one right answer!), but you will benefit from doing what the following questions ask of you. Find answers and think through your responses. Your comfort with these questions will help you as you gather data for all kinds of presentations.

Answer the following questions:

1. Find a quote to support the idea that dogs make better pets than cats. _____

_____

_____

2. Search the Internet to find three resources that give information on how to buy a car. _____

_____

_____

_____

3. Think of a story that would be appropriate for you to tell in a speech about the adjustments a freshman must make during her first month away at college. _____

_____

_____

_____

_____

_____

4. Find an annual report of a major company. (Anyone who owns stock in a company receives these publications in the mail. You can write companies for a copy, or visit a college career center to review annual reports.) Look through the publication to determine:

a. The mission statement of the organization.

b. The names of the Board of Trustees.

c. A letter from the President.

_____

_____

_____

_____

_____

5. Visit your library and learn to use the *Reader's Guide to Periodical Literature*.

6. Conduct a practice interview with someone who has an interesting job. If possible, tie this assignment to another project you've been working on.

7. Find two legitimate sources of statistics that support contradictory points of view.

_____

_____

8. Which search engine searches most of the other search engines in the Internet?

_____

_____

9. What personal experience have you had that would support a speech? Briefly describe the story and identify the topic of the speech.

_____

_____

_____

10. Find the following information:
   a. Who is the mayor of your hometown?

   _____

   b. What is the population?

   _____

   c. Who is the major employer?

   _____

   d. What is the average individual income?

   _____

Part II

Working on Structure

Chapter 5

Presenting Data

Did you know that according to the American Cancer Society, 70.7 cents of every dollar they raise goes to something other than fund raising and management? In fact, 24% goes to research, 16.4% goes to patient services, 17.7% goes to prevention and 12.6% goes to detection and treatment programs.

Got that? I doubt it! When Patrick gave this introduction to his persuasive speech on donating to the American Cancer Society fund raiser, he made several serious errors. First, he started by telling us that some of our gift goes back to fund raising and management, which is seen as a negative and therefore a disincentive to giving for some people. He should place emphasis on all the obviously positive activities our money goes to support. Second, he lost us with a string of statistics. Third, he used no visuals to support his data. Patrick should present his cause the way the American Cancer Society does in its own brochure. "Your American Cancer Society invests 70.7 cents of every dollar raised on cancer research, patient services, education, prevention, detection, and treatment programs." The statement is supported with the chart on the following page:

The text and visual, combined, make a very effective message that is likely to persuade the audience that the dollar each of us sends goes to accomplish something good in the fight against cancer.

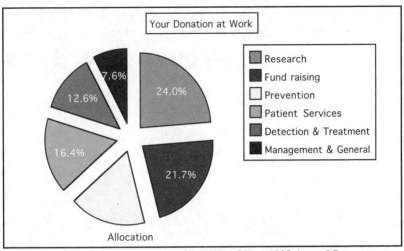

Source: American Cancer Society Combined Fiscal Year 1995 Annual Report.

Including Data Verbally

One guaranteed way to lose the attention of your listeners is to list strings of numbers. When comparing several groups of numerical data, use a visual aid to support your words.

When reciting complicated numbers or statistics, give the exact numbers, then round them off to make them easier to conceptualize.

Example

You may speak about the popularity of a particular television set by discussing sales. You might say that, "There were 501,279 Brand X sets sold last month. Think of it! Over half a million people chose Brand X over all the others on the market."

Sometimes it helps your listeners visualize your meaning if you state statistics several different ways.

Example

If you were giving information about Mt. Everest, you could describe the mountain this way: "Mt. Everest is 29,028 feet tall. At over 29,000 feet, Mt. Everest is the tallest mountain in the world. More than 4,400 people have tried to climb to the top and only 728 have made it. That means that over 85% of those who fight freezing weather, horrible storms, and grueling physical demands never to make it to the summit."

Including Data in Visual Form

Charts and graphs can add meaning to the numbers and lists you include in your presentation. If you have a significant amount of data, a visual can allow the audience to make comparisons and absorb information easily. Deciding which type of visual will most effectively convey your message can be challenging.

Types of Visuals

LISTS

A simple list is often the best way to show information. Every David Letterman fan knows the "Top 10" format. This is a simple list of items. Some lists contain columns of data. According to Ed Castrege of Villanova's University Shop, a list of the topselling textbooks for the 1998 school year looks like this.

Example

	Title	Number Sold
1.	*Holt Handbook*	1,832
2.	*Holy Bible* (New Revised Standard Version)	1,420
3.	*Business Financial Management* (Couley and Heck)	967
4.	*Legal Environment of Business* (Cross)	716
5.	*Understanding Movies* (Gianetti)	532

BAR GRAPHS

Bar graphs are an effective way to compare quantitative data.

Example

A simple bar graph comparing the number of books in the Harvard University Library (13,369,855) versus the Yale University Library (9,758,341) would look like the following graph:

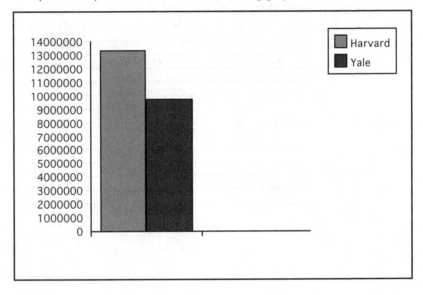

LINE GRAPHS

Line graphs are primarily used to indicate precise changes over time.

Example

A line graph showing enrollment at Wallace University from 1985 to 1995 would look like the graph on the following page:

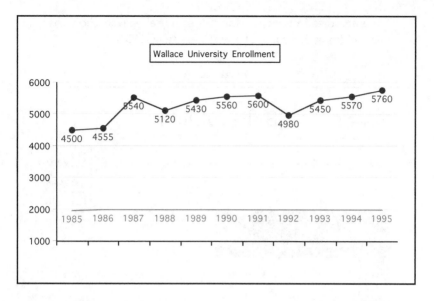

PIE CHARTS

A pie chart is an effective way of showing percentages. The whole pie equals 100% and each slice represents the percentage allocated to that slice.

Example

This data represents the findings of Albert Mehrabian in his 1967 paper titled "Decoding of Inconsistent Communication."

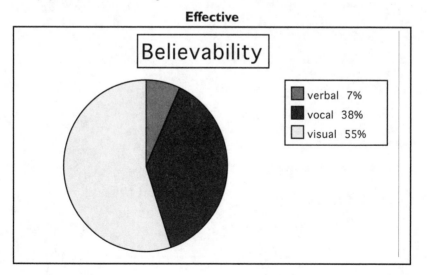

The same data in bar chart form does not effectively show that the selected items are parts of a whole equaling 100%.

Ineffective

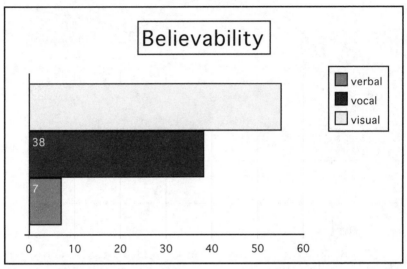

The bar chart is an appropriate way to compare data over time and determine trends.

Example: Visualizing a Trend

Effective

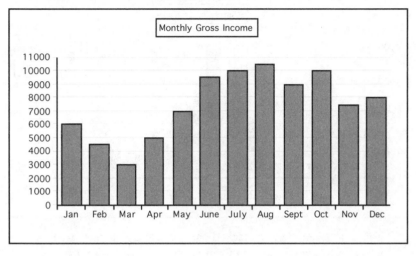

This is the same data in pie chart form. Notice that the data is not easy to read and the trend over time is not clear.

Ineffective

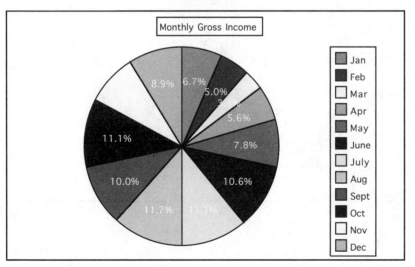

Both the bar chart and area chart allow for easy comparison of data.

Example: Stacked Bar Chart and Stacked Area Chart Using Same Data

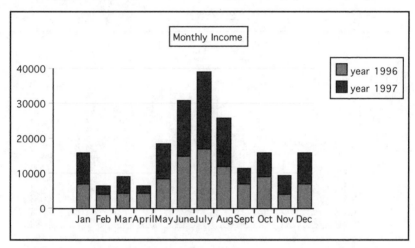

This is an example of a stacked bar chart and a stacked area chart, which in this case add data from one year to the next, giving an easy representation of two years' total income.

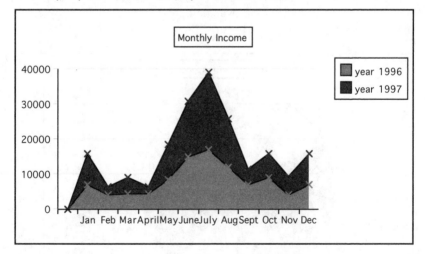

The simple bar chart and line graph do not add data, but display two variables side by side, allowing for easy comparison.

Example: Bar Chart and Line Graph Using Same Data

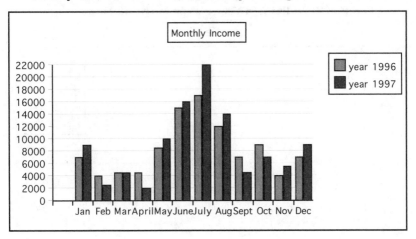

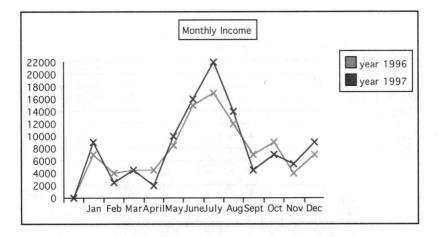

This line graph is ineffective because it shows similar data trends that are hard to distinguish in this format. A standard bar chart is more effective at comparing this data from year to year.

Example: Visualizing a Trend over Multiple Years

Ineffective

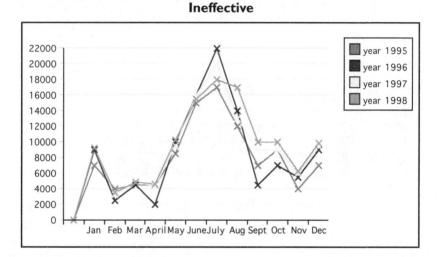

Effective

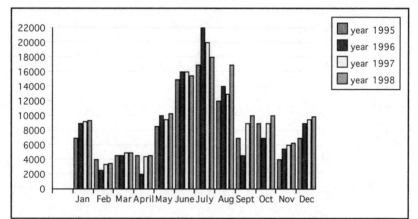

If you would like to see the information from year to year in a four-year total, use a stacked area graph.

Effective

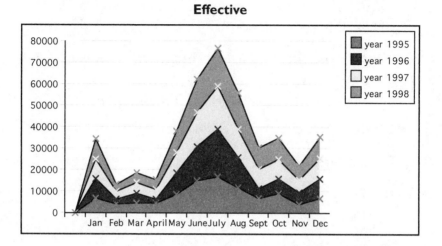

Accurate data is essential to your presentation. How you present data, both verbally and visually, determines the effectiveness of your message.

The following exercises will help you present data effectively.

Exercises

CHOOSING VISUALS

Objective

To become familiar with several ways to visually present data.

Method

Review the ways to present data covered in this chapter. Choose which form of graph or chart best represents the data in each question. Either sketch the charts by hand or create them on a computer.

What type of visual aid would best show the following messages?

1. "New York has more skyscrapers than any other city in the world. New York has 131, Chicago has 47, Hong Kong has 30, Houston has 27 and Los Angeles has 21." (*Source:* "The Top 10 of Everything 1998" by Russell Ash.)

---

2. The family budget is divided into these things:

Rent	$900
First car payment	$255
Second car payment	$380
Food	$500
Utilities	$450
Clothing	$350
Savings	$200
Miscellaneous	?

Total take-home pay is $3,700. What is the percentage of take-home pay for each item and what is the miscellaneous amount?

---

3. How many speeding tickets were issued by Officer Dana compared to tickets issued by Officer Lynne.

Dana:		**Lynne:**	
January	21	January	14
February	19	February	13
March	33	March	34
April	39	April	43
May	55	May	13
June	77	June	53
July	64	July	43
August	97	August	101
September	59	September	81
October	77	October	41
November	45	November	31
December	34	December	19

_____

_____

_____

4. Take the data from question 3 and portray the total tickets given by both officers.

_____

_____

_____

5. Compare the amount your fraternity raised last year on its annual pizza sale ($266.94) to the amount earned over the last two years. (Year 1 = $107.88, Year 2 = $143.03)

_____

_____

_____

The answers are found on the following three pages.

1. A simple list would look like this:

    New York   131
    Chicago   47
    Hong Kong   30
    Houston   27
    Los Angeles   21

    A bar chart would look like this:

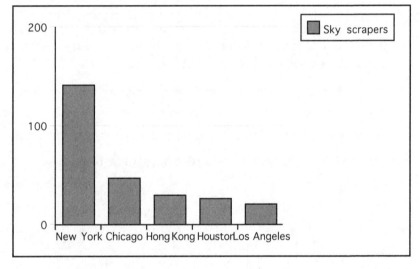

2. A pie chart shows percentages and would look like this for this question:

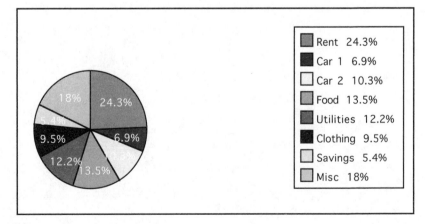

3. A bar chart shows a comparison of the officers' ticket numbers.

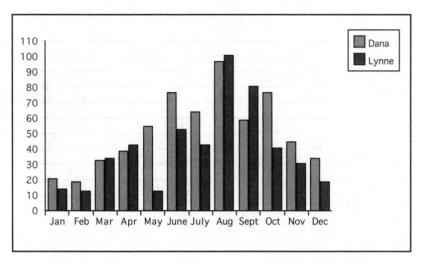

4. The stacked data bar graph combines as well as compares information.

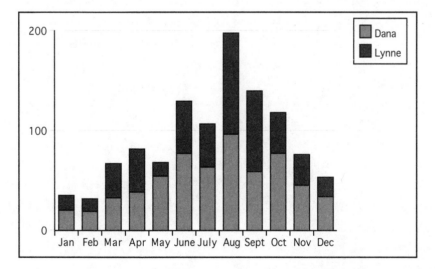

5. A standard bar chart shows your three-year progression.

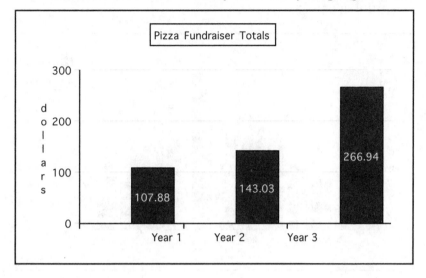

Chapter 6

Organizing Your Information

In "Getting Started," you created a list of ideas and organized them into a loose structure. Once you've got the natural groupings from your list, it's time to organize your points into patterns and then create an outline. The pattern you choose should help the audience make the most sense out of your material. The most widely used organizational patterns are:

- Chronological
- Spatial
- Topical
- Causal
- Problem-solution

Chronological

This pattern organizes information in time sequence. Some of us may remember reading children's stories that began, "Once upon a time. . ." and progressed to ". . . and they lived happily ever after." Those stories were almost always written in a chronological pattern. Demonstrations are given in step-by-step order, as well as presentations that ask us to look at the past, present, and future.

Examples: Topics You Might Organize Chronologically
The history of the Democratic party in the United States

The life of Katherine Hepburn

The best method to build a campfire

Spatial

As you can tell from the root word—space—this pattern is arranged geographically: east to west, north to south, left to right or by location. Many informative speeches are structured in this form.

Examples: Topics You Can Discuss Spatially
How to get to North Face Lodge

The design of the new bookstore

The vineyards of the California wine country.

Topical

This is probably the most frequently used pattern for organizing presentations and is often the easiest to create. The things you'll talk about are organized into categories you create yourself, and they are based on each item's relationship to the topic.

Example: Presentation on New Thought Churches in America
I. Unity

II. Religious Science

III. Christian Science

Example: Eating a Healthy Diet
I. The old food pyramid

II. The new food pyramid

III. Recent discoveries regarding food's antioxidant qualities

Example: Birds of the Eastern Shore of Maryland
I. Waterfowl

II. Songbirds

III. Raptors

Causal

This pattern develops a relationship that shows how the occurrence of one thing is a direct result of another thing.

Example: A Speech on Dental Hygiene

"Tooth decay is influenced by not brushing and flossing, eating sugar, and heredity."

This establishes what effect has occurred.

Your goal might be:

I want the audience to understand how tooth decay occurs.

Your main points might include:

I. Not brushing and flossing leads to cavities.
II. Eating sugar leads to cavities.
III. Heredity can affect tooth decay.

These three main points and appropriate supporting data establish the causes.

Example: The Health Risks of Smoking

I want my audience to understand the relationship between smoking and physical illness. The main points might be:

I. Smoking is directly related to several kinds of cancer.
II. Smoking leads to the onset of heart disease.
III. Smoking is related to diseases of the skin.

When these main points are supported by accurate data, they show that smoking causes illnesses.

Problem-Solution

This pattern is used most often in persuasive speeches and in some technical briefings. The structure describes an existing problem, gives reasons for the solution, states potential solutions, and points out your recommended action.

Examples

Contributing to Habitat for Humanity can change lives.

Raising tuition only 4% will increase the number of services students receive.

The new drug to prevent prostate cancer is ready for release.

Once you have chosen the problem-solution pattern, try to anticipate the questions your audience will generate.

Answer as many questions as possible when you develop the presentation. Be prepared to answer any questions you don't address in a question-and-answer period.

Tip: Use the problem-solution format for adult learners. They become involved in this type of format.

The following exercises will help you organize your information.

Exercises

CHOOSING APPROPRIATE PATTERNS OF ORGANIZATION

Objective

To choose appropriate patterns of organization based on the topic and setting.

Method

In the space provided, identify the *pattern* you would use for each topic. Include your *reasons* for selecting it. Choose from these patterns:

Chronological
Spatial
Topical
Causal
Problem-solution

1. A description of your vacation to London. _____

   _____

   _____

2. Why better recycling programs are needed in your community. _____

   _____

   _____

3. How to get from the Phoenix airport to the Phoenician conference center. _____

   _____

   _____

4. The health issues associated with smoking. _____

5. Ways to create interest in a training program._____

6. Opening a new dance studio. _____

7. Hiking the Appalachian Trail. _____

8. Painting a house for profit. _____

9. Why to buy tires designed for driving on wet roads.__

10. Explain how to make chocolate chip cookies._____

The answers are found on the following two pages.

ANSWERS

1. **A description of your vacation to London.** This could be done using a chronological pattern if you described the events of each day sequentially. The vacation could also be described spatially if you traveled from east to west, north to south, etc. A topical pattern could be used by dividing the topic into categories like historical sites, night life, and shopping.

2. **Why better recycling programs are needed in your community.** A problem-solution pattern would probably be the best pattern for this persuasive presentation.

3. **How to get from the Phoenix airport to the Phoenician conference center.** This involves giving directions, which is best done spatially.

4. **The health issues associated with smoking.** A cause-and-effect pattern would be the most effective approach, listing statistics that link smoking to cancer, heart problems, and other health problems.

5. **Ways to create interest in a training program.** This topic could best be approached with a topical pattern.

6. **Opening a new dance studio.** Using a sequential approach might be the most appropriate way to speak about opening any new business. A topical pattern would also be an acceptable method, organizing information into categories like finances, location, marketing, personnel, etc.

7. **Hiking the Appalachian Trail.** This would be an appropriate topic to discuss spatially. The trail could be traced from south to north or in sections by state or region.

8. **Painting a house for profit.** This presentation could be designed in a chronological style, starting with the estimate and bid process and progressing through the completion of the job and receipt of the final check.

9. **Why your audience should buy tires designed for driving on wet roads.** A problem-solution approach to persuasion would be an effective method of convincing the audience that driving on wet weather tires can prevent accidents.

10. **How to make chocolate chip cookies.** Directions should be given in a sequential, chronological pattern.

Chapter 7

Introductions

You have the most power to make an impact on your audience at the beginning and the end of your presentation.

In the beginning, the audience is fresh and, for the most part, open to your message. Most audiences want you to present with confidence and poise. Most audiences make up their minds about your credibility within the first three minutes of hearing your introduction. Consequently, your introduction is critical to your success. The beginning of your presentation should meet the following criteria.

Introduction Goals

IT'S RELEVANT TO YOUR TOPIC.

The introduction must relate to your message in content, tone, and style. An interesting story that gets our attention and has an impact is *not* an appropriate attention getter if it bears no relevance to the content of the speech. A humorous story of your trip to the auditorium that morning may not be a good opener if it has nothing to do with your presentation. Choose something that supports, illuminates, or illustrates your message.

IT CREATES A POSITIVE RELATIONSHIP.

Establish a positive relationship with your audience by letting them know, "We're in this thing together. I'm not here to antagonize you, turn you off by my superior knowledge, or make you feel uncomfortable." You can build a positive relationship by:

- Choosing strong, but not offensive words.
- Using an appropriate tone of voice.
- Even if your opinions contradict those of the audience, letting them know that you respect them.

IT GETS THE AUDIENCE INVOLVED.

The introduction should welcome the audience to your message and get each member thinking about how the presentation relates to them personally. They will ask the famous question, "What's in it for me?" They will wonder if it's worth their effort to listen. A good introduction will answer with, "There's a lot in it for you! Just listen to what's coming."

IT GETS ATTENTION.

It's important to "hook" your audience into paying attention right away. Plan the first words you utter carefully to get your listeners to "perk up their ears" and listen for what's coming next. You won't get another chance to make that first impression; so you'll want to do everything possible to do it right the first time. If your listeners aren't involved from the beginning, it's especially challenging to get them interested in the middle.

Techniques That Get Attention

USE AN ANECDOTE OR TELL A BRIEF STORY.

Use a good story as an effective way to make a point. An anecdote can illustrate your real message and makes the message "real" to your listeners. If you have several stories you'd like to tell in your presentation, it's sometimes a good idea to use the best one as your introduction.

We all know someone who can tell a great story. We also know people who just can't. Make sure you're in the first group if you choose this approach! If you're not sure, ask your friends. Practice telling your story before a group who will not be attending your presentation. Choose a group similar to the makeup of your audience for your practice. Adapt it according to their reactions.

Caution: Even if you're an expert storyteller, don't use foul language or tell an off-color story. You cannot recover from this mistake.

ESTABLISH COMMON GROUND.

You can damage your credibility as an information source if the audience members feel you couldn't possibly relate to them.

Example

Imagine yourself in this situation: The speaker was asked to fill in at the last minute and knew nothing about the audience. She had less than 24 hours to prepare a seminar on stress management for an audience of 30 people. Having spoken on this topic before, she quickly prepared information and, on the morning of the speech, she entered the room with confidence.

The room she entered was a lunchroom filled with 30 middle-aged, male, blue-collar workers who had just gotten off the 11 P.M.–7 A.M. shift. They were forced to go to this monthly safety meeting but wanted to go home. Our speaker, having prepared for an executive breakfast was wearing a three-piece suit and high-heeled pumps; she was carrying an expensive leather briefcase. She knew that to have any credibility with her audience she had to change the introduction to her speech and immediately establish some relationship with them.

After she was introduced, she walked to the front of the room and rather than stand behind the table, she sat on top of it, crossing her ankles. She began the presentation this way:

> Shift work is usually hard, dirty and stressful. For eight years I was married to a cop who changed shifts every five days. We almost never had a normal meal or a good night's sleep. We had no social life—people wouldn't call or ask us out because he was always sleeping or at work. I spent a lot of time alone. You may have noticed that I said I *was* married to a cop. We divorced two years ago. Yeah, shift work is stressful.

By using this anecdote, the speaker salvaged a potential disaster. The audience perked up, shared common stories, and listened to her suggestions.

REFER TO A PREVIOUS SPEAKER.

This technique works because of timing and relevance. It lets the audience know you paid attention to the same thing they did. (And if they weren't paying attention, it let them know what they missed and that you found it important.) You have the opportunity to tie together the theme of the day. Your comment has to be sincere; misquoting the previous speaker or mispronouncing her name can turn everyone off.

ASK A QUESTION.

In just a few quick words, a good question asked in your introduction can not only gain the attention of the audience, but also can focus them on your topic and relate it to themselves. Usually the question is rhetorical, one you don't expect anyone to answer out loud. If you would like a response, let the audience know. For a small audience (30 or less), you can ask for speakers to call out answers. Ask larger groups for a show of hands.

A good question can also set the tone of the presentation.

Examples
For a presentation on cystic fibrosis, one speaker began with a series of questions:

"Have you ever had a bad cold that made you cough constantly?

Have you ever had a cough that made you feel exhausted when you could finally get your breath?

Have you ever coughed so hard you didn't know if you could even get your next breath?

Well, that's what every morning is like for Steve Sanders."

Another speaker told the story of a family nearly destroyed by how they reacted to winning the lottery by asking, "How much money is too much?"

Both of these examples show that often an opening question is combined with a story related to the question. The question itself is usually not sufficient to stand alone as an introduction. Combine the question with another opening technique.

MAKE A BOLD STATEMENT.

Examples

"In only four seconds, thousands of people saw their lives turn to rubble. Ninety five hundred died. The force was the equivalent of five atomic bombs." This was the introduction to a speech on the power of earthquakes. The speaker chose to use the powerful Mexico City earthquake, which rated 7.9 on the Richter scale, to get the attention of the audience.

A startling statistic works just as well.

Example

Four out of ten Americans will be the victim of a crime this year.

USE HUMOR.

Starting your presentation with a laugh can help establish a friendly relationship with your audience. Generally, the more original the humor, the better. If you are naturally funny and possess a good sense of timing, relating your own story to the topic might work. Make sure that, if you choose to use humor, it is appropriate for your topic. For instance, don't start a presentation on breast cancer prevention with a laugh.

Using a canned joke presents certain dangers: The audience may have heard the story. It's very hard to recover from the sinking feeling that comes from hearing your audience pretend to laugh at your joke. If your humor bombs, move on quickly. Explaining or belaboring a bad joke just makes it worse. Apologizing works only if it's quick, simple, and straightforward. A long apology simply makes the audience more uncomfortable. Obviously, avoid using any language or making any references that could offend your listeners.

GIVE A DEFINITION.

Example

"'Abandoned . . . given up; forsaken; deserted.' That's the way *Webster's New World College Dictionary* defines the word. I would define it as three months alone in the darkness." That is the way Lynne Peterson began her presentation on spending a cold winter alone in rural Alaska.

Choose a word that creates a visual image of the tone you want your presentation to portray. If you quote a specific dictionary, reference the source.

MAKE A HISTORICAL REFERENCE.

Starting your talk with a reference to an event related to your topic draws the audience into your presentation. Some presentations open with an event that occurred that day or that week in history. Every day is the anniversary of something. Many sources list the dates of historical events. You can find resources in libraries, local newspapers, and the Internet.

You may choose historical events that relate to your topic regardless of the exact day of their occurrence.

Example
It might be appropriate to open with a reference to the Challenger explosion for presentations on the contribution of teachers in the United States, how a lack of communication can have disastrous results, or the permanent impact visual stimuli has on us.

USE A PROP OR GIMMICK.

Introductions using the unexpected provide excellent attention getters.

Example
Beginning your presentation in complete silence while signing your introduction in American sign language would be dramatic.

Attention getting is a good thing, but doing dangerous or illegal things is not!

Examples
Taking out a dollar bill, lighting it, and watching it burn without saying a word grabs the attention of your audience as you begin to talk about waste in the corporate budget.

Lighting a firecracker as an introduction to a presentation on American holidays is a third.

Burning money (which is illegal) and lighting firecrackers (which is dangerous and sometimes illegal) are *not recommended* attention getters.

Example

The speaker assumed his position at the front of the room. Before he said a word, someone turned out all the lights in the room. He began by saying, "On November 9, 1965, the lights went out in New York City." He continued to tell the story of the first major blackout in United States history. At the end of his introduction, someone turned the lights on and he began the body of his speech on power usage in the United States.

Caution: Even this introduction has a dangerous quality. The speaker was sure to check that everyone was seated and no one else was entering the room when he began speaking in the dark.

GIVE A QUOTE.

A thought-provoking quote can provide an excellent start for your speech. People like to know what famous or high-ranking people have to say. You can piggyback on the credibility of the person you quote if you carefully craft your introduction around the words of a well-respected source. With all the resources available today, you can find quotes on any subject. Bookstores, the library, and the Internet store a multitude of sources for quotations. Try to quote someone who has credibility with your audience.

When you use a quote, choose a brief and concise one. Paraphrase the parts you feel are insignificant to the "meat" of what you want to express, while maintaining the intended message of the statement.

Examples: Quotes in Introductions

"A man of my spiritual intensity does not eat corpses." This is a George Bernard Shaw quote used to begin a powerful presentation on the dangers of eating meat in an age of bacteria and disease-carrying animal products. (The *Concise Columbia Dictionary of Quotations*)

To begin an acceptance speech for science teacher of the year, Joanna used this quote from *The Little Zen Companion*:

"There is a Chinese proverb which goes like this, 'Teachers open the door, but you must enter by yourself.' In fourth grade, Mrs. Barry opened the door for me, which allowed me to enter the amazing world of learning about nature."

Practice exercises are located at the end of the next chapter.

Chapter 8

Conclusions

As we mentioned in the chapter on introductions, you have the most power to make an impact on your audience at the beginning and the end of your presentation.

Your conclusion is usually the last thing the audience hears from you. Since people tend to remember the last things they hear, make sure you conclude carefully and with emphasis.

Conclusion Goals

IT PROVIDES CLOSURE.

A conclusion that trails off can diminish all the good you have done in the body of your speech. Make sure you've covered all the points you intended to address and then conclude with conviction. A good conclusion assures that everyone knows you're finished with the formal part of your time on stage. When you've reached the end of your conclusion, stop!

IT HELPS THE AUDIENCE REMEMBER.

Your conclusion allows you one final opportunity to reemphasize your points. This is the time to remind the audience of what's important. You can repeat the points in a new way to make them more memorable.

IT CAN CALL THE AUDIENCE TO ACTION.

For any persuasive speech, the point of speaking at all is to persuade the audience to do, to think, or to feel something. Just like a salesperson who has a good product to sell, you can do all the convincing in the world, but until you ask them to buy, you haven't finished your job.

Techniques for Conclusions

SUMMARIZE YOUR POINTS.

Most presenters summarize at some point, in either the conclusion or the transition from the last point into the conclusion. Sometimes a summary can simply consist of repeating your main points.

Example: End of a Demonstration Speech on How to Putt
So remember, it's not a complicated process. Just six simple steps can lead you to a lower score:

First, Balance your weight evenly on both feet.

Second, hold your head directly above the ball.

Third, keep your eyes on the ball.

Fourth, keep your elbows locked.

Fifth, use a smooth movement on your backswing and follow through.

Sixth, now sink that putt!

The most common method of summarizing is to make a general statement about your main points.

Example: Conclusion of a Celebratory Speech
And so, you now know how Helen grew from a timid little girl from Omaha to the first CEO of our company. Congratulations, Helen!

REMIND THEM OF WHY IT'S IMPORTANT TO THEM.

In this ending, you'll want to tie the points you've made to the audience's situation. In the chapter on introductions, one of the purposes listed was to get the audience involved. This type of conclusion again answers the question, "What's in it for me?" and gets them involved emotionally.

Example
In introducing a new company procedure for cost cutting, the CEO ended this way: "The new J and J process will mean more work for us, especially until we get used to the changes. In the long run, however, our processing will be more efficient and your work will flow

more smoothly. The bottom line is that the *company's* bottom line will increase, our jobs will become more indispensable, and your profit-sharing bonuses can be even higher than last year!"

ASK THE AUDIENCE TO DO SOMETHING.

This conclusion challenges your listeners to take action. You may be asking them to vote for your candidate, choose your proposal over the others, recycle, or even call their mother! You miss the mark in a persuasive presentation by spending precious time convincing the audience of all the good reasons to do something—and then neglecting to ask them to do it.

Example
The most famous persuasive conclusion is probably that of John F. Kennedy: "Ask not what your country can do for you, ask what you can do for your country."

REFER TO YOUR INTRODUCTION.

This method of concluding brings a presentation full circle. The intro and conclusion meet in the memories of the listeners.

Example
In the "Introduction" chapter, the following introduction was used:

> Shift work is usually hard, dirty and stressful. For eight years I was married to a cop who changed shifts every five days. We almost never had a normal meal or a good night's sleep. We had no social life—people wouldn't call or ask us out because he was always sleeping or at work. I spent a lot of time alone. You may have noticed that I said I *was* married to a cop. We divorced two years ago. Yeah, shift work is stressful.

This introduction and the presentation that followed present a good opportunity to return to the introduction to conclude. Here's one possibility:

Example
> We've covered a lot of techniques for reducing the stress of shift work today. I hope, if you can apply even a few of them, that you will have a different result than I did—that your marriage is strong, and your personal life is *yours*, not your job's.

ANSWER THE QUESTION YOU ASKED IN YOUR INTRODUCTION.

This conclusion also ties the speech together.

Examples

A presentation for supervisors of a major company began with the question, "What do you think that employees in America list as the number one thing that motivates them on the job?" It might end with this conclusion:

> So, as you've seen, the thing people want most from their jobs is not what supervisors think they want. People don't list money or job security at the top of the list of most desired things. The thing employees want most is full appreciation for a job well done! Simply treating people with consideration and honestly appreciating what they do are the best motivators of all. When you go back to work tomorrow, give yourself a checkup to determine how well you provide your employees with what they need.

USE A QUOTE OR RECITE A POEM.

A well-chosen quote or poem can be thought-provoking for your audience. Make sure you choose something that is relevant to your topic and that resonates with the listeners.

Example

A career management consultant ended her presentation, "Balancing Family and Career," for an audience of Christian executive mothers with this Bible quote: "Six days you shall do your work, but on the seventh day you shall rest . . ." (*Exodus* 23:12). Effective and credible!

ENVISION THE FUTURE.

When your presentation involves the future, take the audience ahead to see what might await them.

Example

This brings us to the state of violence in America today. And tomorrow . . . well, the future is up to you. If each and every one of us does one thing to stop the violence—not supporting violent movies, teaching children passive resistance, keeping our environment weapon-free—we can live in a better world. Children will go to schools with no metal detectors, people of all nations will talk, not fight and newspapers will be filled with stories of *good* acts!

Be careful of envisioning a negative future. This can be exceptionally effective as an ending. But it can also fail miserably by depressing your audience and erasing the positive message as well as damaging the positive personal relationship you've developed during the speech. If you choose to see a negative future, make sure that you give your audience a way to improve the situation.

Learn effective endings in the following exercises.

Exercises

Because introductions and conclusions are intrinsically related, the exercises for both topics have been combined in this chapter. Practice your introduction and conclusion at the same time to check for consistency in tone and content. Remember that the beginning and ending of the presentation are the most powerful times you have for "hooking" your audience into your idea.

EFFECTIVE ENDINGS

Objectives

To identify good introductions and conclusions and those that need improvement.

To suggest appropriate changes.

Method

Read each of the following introductions and conclusions, and determine its effectiveness. If it isn't interesting and compelling, determine how and why to improve it.

Introduction Example
Today I'm going to tell you about Bonnie and Clyde.

Improvements
Clyde was a bad guy—a very bad guy. At the same time he was likable—very likable. That's how Bonnie got involved with the man who gave her the time of her life—and death!

Conclusion Example
Today I've gone over the three main steps you can take to protect your car from being stolen. Keep them in mind the next time you go to the mall!

Improvements

Today I've gone over the three main steps you can take to protect your car from being stolen. First, park in an open, well lighted place. Next, notice and remember any suspicious-looking people or vehicles when you park. And finally, lock your doors! Keep these things in mind the next time you go to the mall and chances are your car will be waiting for you when you come out!

Now you're on your own!

Introductions

1. The first step in choosing a computer system is to do your homework on the kinds available.

   Improvements: _____

   _____

   _____

   _____

   _____

2. I want you to remember this: One of us in this room won't make it to age 50 because of a drunk driving accident.

   Improvements: _____

   _____

   _____

   _____

   _____

3. Do you like your job? Most Americans answer "no" to this question. When you consider that job unhappiness is a leading factor in heart disease, you may want to reconsider your answer.

   Improvements: _____

   _____

   _____

   _____

_____

4. Before I start today, I just want to apologize for my scratchy voice.

   Improvements: _____

   _____

   _____

   _____

   _____

5. I want to add something to what Bob just said in his presentation. The figure of two-thirds is not quite right. It's more like three-quarters.

   Improvements: _____

   _____

   _____

   _____

   _____

Conclusions

1. I've explained in detail the new engineering process for the North Face project. Are there any questions?

   Improvements: _____

   _____

   _____

   _____

   _____

2. Today we've looked at the reasons for changing our meal plan. First, it will allow student athletes who have practice during currently scheduled dining hours to be able to have dinner without incurring added expense. Second, it allows dining service workers to have flexible working

hours. And third, the change will eliminate some of the food waste we now have at our university. Please vote yes to changing our meal plan at the student center today!

Improvements: _____

_____

_____

_____

_____

3. So those are some important facts about the life of Dan Rather. Thank you.

Improvements: _____

_____

_____

_____

_____

4. Picture yourself free of carrying keys, credit cards, drivers license, membership cards, even cash. Imagine being able to go out to dinner, to the movies, even on a vacation without carrying a wallet or purse! That's what our future looks like when the "Eyedentification" program is in effect. You can be unencumbered!

Improvements: _____

_____

_____

_____

_____

5. Thank you for letting me tell you about my experiences snow boarding on Mount Hood. I guess that's about it.

Improvements: _____

_____

_____

TECHNIQUES THAT WORK

Objective

To learn by observation, which introduction and conclusion techniques work most effectively.

Method

At various times, over several days, tune your cable TV to the C-Span channel. This channel televises speeches and discussions of national political interest. Watch several different types of presentations, paying special attention to the beginning and ending of each. Observe the following:

1. Was the introduction relevant to the topic?
2. Did the speaker establish a positive relationship?
3. Was the audience encouraged to get involved intellectually? Emotionally?
4. Which techniques did the speaker use to gain attention?
5. Was the conclusion relevant to the topic?
6. Which technique did the speaker use to conclude the presentation?
7. If the speaker were to start over again with this presentation, what suggestions would you make regarding the introduction and conclusion to make the presentation even more effective?

TYING THINGS TOGETHER

Objectives

To become comfortable with a variety of techniques for opening and closing presentations.

To choose appropriate opening and closing statements.

To choose introductions and conclusions that compliment each other.

Method

You have been asked to speak on the following list of topics. Think through the requirements for appropriate introductions and conclusions, and decide on at least two introductions and conclusions you might use for each topic.

- Save Social Security
- The kickoff for a new sales campaign for your favorite company
- Comparison of two good computer systems
- The need for creative thinking
- How to set up a new aquarium
- The life of Martin Luther King
- Opening a bed and breakfast
- Painting with watercolor
- Financing your first home
- Using humor in presentations

Example: Kayaking the Fjords of Alaska

Introduction. Imagine yourself on a sunny day, skimming along blue waters, smooth as glass. You're surrounded by mountains and glaciers, and the smell of pine permeates the air. Suddenly you hear a burst of water and see a shiny black arch appear on the surface. Immediately you realize you're kayaking with the magnificent orcas....

Conclusion. So the next time you're choosing a vacation site, consider Alaska where the exhilaration of kayaking with the orcas is almost as common as walking your dog.

Chapter 9

Outlining

Now that you have gathered and organized the ideas for your speech, it's time to refine the list into an outline. Even if you think you'll skip this step and work from your groupings—*don't*. An outline is essential to the success of your speech.

Think of your outline as a road map. Yes, you can get from point A to point B without using a map. You may have to visit a few other points and stop to ask for directions once or twice, but you'll eventually get there. When you give a speech, you can't afford to wander from place to place. Your audience will not continue to listen if you frequently digress. You must move efficiently, effectively, and logically from point A to point B. Your outline helps you to do that.

The outline also can provide a good psychological boost. Knowing the exact points in the precise order you'll give them can make you feel more comfortable and well prepared.

Outline Format Rules

BE CONSISTENT.

Formal outlines follow a specific set of rules.

Example: A Basic Format
I. Main point: This is usually indicated by Roman numerals.

   A. Major divisions of the main point are indented and indicated by capital letters.

   1. Minor subdivisions are indicated by Arabic numerals and are further indented.

   2. Continue until you've listed all your minor subdivisions.

  B. Second major subdivision.

II. Second main point

  A. Second major division

   1. Subdivision 1

   2. Subdivision 2

Since it's a universal practice to use this format, it's good to be familiar with it and use it consistently.

MATCH As WITH Bs, 1s WITH 2s.

For each supporting point, you need at least one other supporting point. It seems silly to point out, but you can't divide a point into parts if there is only one part. The reason for subordinating points is to separate ideas.

Example

I. The legal drinking age should be raised to 21.

  A. The legal voting age is 21.

II. . . .

In this example, having only one point does not support the premise sufficiently for you to make your argument. At least two subpoints should be listed:

Example

I. The legal drinking age should be raised to 21.

  A. The legal voting age is 21.

  B. Insurance statistics show a significant decrease in accidents after age 21.

II. . . .

This example supports your premise in two categories.

USE COMPLETE SENTENCES.

As tempting as it may be to use short phrases for your outline, you'll find it beneficial to use full sentences during the road map phase. A full sentence lets you see if you truly meet your goals in clearly stating and supporting your main points.

Example

Compare these two statements of a specific point. Which would you find more effective?

I. The history of our company.

II. Our company grew in three distinct stages.

The second is more effective because it clearly signals exactly what you will say in this section.

Reminder: This is your outline, not a script or your speaker notes. This is the road map you'll use to navigate. A good outline might be about one-fourth the number of words as your script.

LIST ONLY ONE POINT WITH EACH SYMBOL.

Don't combine ideas within a point. List ideas separately to keep them clear in your own mind and to develop each individually.

Example

Compare the following two subpoint strategies:

A. Dancing offers physical, psychological, and emotional benefits.

B. Partner dancing offers three main benefits:

  1. The physical benefits of dancing include a good cardiovascular workout.

  2. The social outlet provided by being able to dance provides a strong psychological benefit.

  3. Partner dancing is an excellent opportunity to spend time with the special person in your life, which offers excellent emotional benefits.

Option B is more clear and specific.

USE BETWEEN TWO AND FIVE MAIN POINTS.

Your audience will find more than five main points confusing and hard to remember. Speakers often choose three main points because groupings of three are easy to remember. Make sure your main points are mutually exclusive.

INCLUDE ALL SECTIONS.

List the specific purpose, thesis statement, and resources on the outline. Even though these things aren't included in the actual speech presentation, listing them on the outline facilitates identification of any structural problems.

WRITE OUT TRANSITIONAL PHRASES.

The wording used to move the listener from one point into the next is important to the flow of the presentation. Write out the full sentence you will use between main points.

WRITE OUT THE INTRODUCTION AND CONCLUSION.

Insert the introduction and conclusion where they will appear in the formal speech. Use the format options listed in the "Introductions" and "Conclusions" chapters.

Practice your outlining skills in the following exercise.

Exercises

SCRAMBLED MESSAGE

Objective

To correctly structure an outline.

Method

The following is an outline of a presentation of how to prepare an informative speech. Read each line carefully and rearrange the statements to form a logical outline. Each line is numbered for your reference in rearranging the lines.

(Thanks to Cecile Blanche of Villanova University for providing this example.)

Sample outline for informative speech

1. I. INTRODUCTION
2. II. BODY/DISCUSSION
3. III. CONCLUSION
4. THESIS: Careful preparation and successful public speaking go hand in hand.
5. References
6. Professional publications and manuals may be helpful.
7. Use your textbook for reference.

8. After you finish the outline for your speech, you will need to put your speaker's notes on index cards.
9. Let us now review what we have said in this brief space.
10. Interview: C.S. Blanche, Professor of Public Speaking.
11. Research can begin in the library, but this campus is rich in other resources.
12. Pick one that is familiar to you and that you find interesting.
13. Check to see if what you already know can suggest two or three main points that you want to expand.
14. Consult handout papers for advice.
15. Would you take the time to prepare carefully?
16. Write down all that you know about the topic.
17. All great speakers practice aloud.
18. Campus experts are easily accessible.
19. Try to determine what kind of material you need to find.
20. Now that you have laid the groundwork, you are ready to begin your research.
21. Try practicing while looking into a mirror or before a video camera.
22. Don't overlook the Internet as a possible source.
23. How would you like to get an A on your speech?
24. Interviewing experts may be a rewarding experience as well as a rich source of information.
25. Careful preparation and successful public speaking go hand in hand.
26. Community experts (politicians, police, etc.) can be helpful.
27. Up to now we have been talking about finding material, now let us move on to arranging this material into a logical sequence.
28. Osborne and Osborne, *Public Speaking* (New York: Houghten Mifflin, 1992).
29. Begin to work on the body of your speech and move on to the conclusion and then the introduction.
30. Practice is essential to smooth delivery style.
31. Choose a pattern of organization and select the main points.
32. You will then need to use supporting material to develop these points.
33. The first order of business is to choose a topic.
34. S. Brydon and M. Scott, *Between One and Many* (CA: Mayfield, 1994).
35. Consult the *Reader's Guide* for current sources on your topic.
36. Let us turn now to the steps involved in careful preparation.

Hint: Transitional phrases are indented.

ANSWER

SAMPLE OUTLINE FOR INFORMATIVE SPEECH

1. I. INTRODUCTION
23.   A. How would you like to get an A on your speech?
15.   B. Would you take the time to prepare carefully?
7.   1. Use your textbook for reference.
14.   2. Consult handout papers for advice.
4. THESIS: Careful preparation and successful public speaking go hand in hand.
36. Let us turn now to the steps involved in careful preparation.
2. II. BODY/DISCUSSION
33.   A. The first order of business is to choose a topic.
12.   1. Pick one that is familiar to you and that you find interesting.
16.   2. Write down all that you know about the topic.
13.   a. Check to see if what you already know can suggest two or three main points that you want to expand.
19.   b. Try to determine what kind of material you need to find.
20. Now that you have laid the groundwork you are ready to begin your research.
11.   B. Research can begin in the library, but this campus is rich in other resources.
35.   1. Consult the *Reader's Guide* for current sources on your topic.
22.   a. Don't overlook the Internet as a possible source.
6.   b. Professional publications and manuals may be helpful.
24.   2. Interviewing experts may be a rewarding experience as well as a rich source of information.
18.   a. Campus experts are easily accessible.
26.   b. Community experts (politicians, police, etc.) can be helpful.
27. Up to now we have been talking about finding material, now let us move on to arranging this material into a logical sequence.
29.   C. Begin to work on the body of your speech and move on to the conclusion and then the introduction.

31.   1. Choose a pattern of organization and select the
        main points.
32.   2. You will then need to use supporting material to
        develop these points.
 8.   3. After you finish the outline for your speech you will
        need to put your speaker's notes on index cards.
17.   a. All great speakers practice aloud.
21.   b. Try practicing while looking into a mirror or
           before a video camera.
27. Let us now review what we have said in this brief space.
33. III. CONCLUSION
25.   A. Careful preparation and successful public speaking go
        hand in hand.
30.   B. Practice is essential to smooth delivery style.
 5. References
28. Osborne and Osborne, *Public Speaking* (New York: Houghten
    Mifflin, 1992).
34. S. Brydon and M. Scott, *Between One and Many* (CA: Mayfield,
    1994).
10. Interview: C.S. Blanche Professor of Public Speaking.

Part III

Delivering Your Message

Chapter 10

Physical Environment

The room arrangement, room size, lighting, extrinsic noise, as well as temperature and air flow all affect your presentation. Good planning helps you to exercise control over these outside influences.

Room Arrangement

Chairs, tables, and desks are normally set in four basic arrangements. Each has unique requirements to make the best use of your presentation time.

CLASSROOM STYLE

This is the style most commonly used for small to medium-sized public speaking situations requiring one primary speaker or a panel of speakers. Classroom style is a moderately formal arrangement and can look like this:

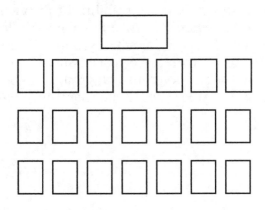

THEATER STYLE

Nearly every large, formal speaking situation uses this seating arrangement. An audience of over 100 is seated this way to allow for more space in the room. Formal, bolted, or hooked chairs allow for limited interaction between audience members, and therefore this arrangement is not recommended for training situations. Theater style looks like this:

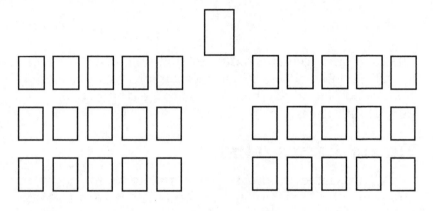

U-SHAPED

This arrangement is conducive for a small group of 25 or less and is effective for training settings. The trainer can walk into the middle of the "U" and interact directly with each participant. Participants can make eye contact with most other members of the group, allowing for interaction among the audience members as well as with the speaker.

A disadvantage is the possibility of distraction, which might be caused when audience members can look at each other. The limited space for small group discussions is also challenging. To overcome the space issue, move chairs into the middle of the "U" so that small groups can be formed on both sides of the table. The "U shape arrangement looks like this:

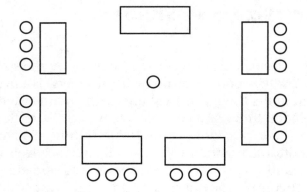

CONFERENCE STYLE

Many presentations that require small group discussions are arranged in conference style. Participants can interact easily and have a work space where they can take notes, handle other papers, or view three-dimensional objects. Many after-dinner speakers find themselves using this arrangement. The disadvantages include numerous distractions as well as discomfort for some audiences members who must turn either their body or chair to see the speaker. This is a conference style:

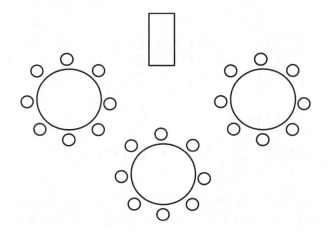

Room Size and Shape

The atmosphere you create is affected by the size of the room. A small room, crowded with listeners, is uncomfortable and limits the speaker's ability to maintain attention for an extended time. Audience members become restless more quickly than in a more comfortable setting. Conversely, a large auditorium setting with a small audience feels uncomfortable and cold to both the speaker and audience. Some may feel conspicuous in this setting and want to "slip out the back." If you find yourself in this situation, ask everyone in the auditorium to move to the front. People hate to do this, but once they have settled into a new seat, they regain their comfort level.

SHAPE

Long, narrow rooms present a challenge for the speaker. Ideally, the speaker is able to move as she speaks in this setting. If this is not possible, the best choice is to stand in the middle of the long side of the room:

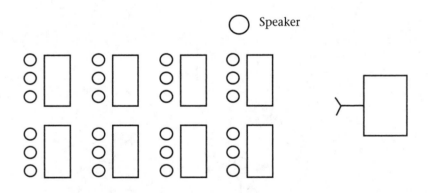

If slides are shown, the screen should be placed on the narrow end of the room and the speaker must adapt, moving from long wall (for best eye contact) to short wall (to gesture to visual aids and change slides).

LIGHTING

Stage lights should illuminate the speaker's face. This means that at least one light must be placed at the speaker's eye level or below. Most rooms are equipped with only overhead fluorescent lights, which cause the speaker's face to "wash out." Features become dark and indistinct. Request extra lighting when possible.

House lights are those above the audience. If the audience must take notes or interact with each other, the house lights should be sufficient for them to see well. Formal speaking situations demand dim house lights, focusing attention on the speaker.

NOISE

Extrinsic noise is distracting and damages a presentation.

Example
A panel discussion was held in an auditorium at the same time a formal recognition dinner was taking place. The only space separating the dining room and the auditorium was the kitchen. The large dining room was acoustically designed to eliminate noise from the kitchen. Unfortunately, because the auditorium and kitchen were considered unrelated, the architects did not consider the effects of kitchen noises on the auditorium. Neither the panel members nor the audience could hear well because of kitchen noises.

Good preparation can eliminate potential problems. Check for internal room noise caused by electrical equipment or audience members. External noises are caused by concurrent events in adjacent rooms, workers making repairs, fire engines, etc. Check the noise conditions at several times of the day to avoid potential problems.

TEMPERATURE AND AIR FLOW

The room should be about 68 degrees. Warmer settings encourage sleepiness. Cooler settings are comfortable for some but distract those not dressed appropriately. Err on the side of cool temperatures!

A gentle air flow that doesn't blow directly on anyone is ideal. A stuffy room induces claustrophobia and mental dullness.

The Ideal Setting

The ideal situation for a *training* session includes one chair (with a hard surface for writing) for everyone in the group and a moderate amount of available space for small group activities. Everyone should be able to see visuals clearly, and the trainer should easily make eye contact with all participants.

For a *public speaking* situation, use a room large enough for all audience members to sit comfortably and see the speaker. There should be few empty chairs, and the room should be comfortably cool.

Increase your awareness of the physical environment in the following exercise.

Exercises

NOISE

Objectives

To become consciously aware of the noises that can interfere with a presentation.

To become aware of methods to effectively deal with noise when speaking.

Method

Attend several presentations given by different speakers in different settings. Make sure to include the room in which you will eventually speak. Listen not to the words the speaker is saying, but to all the extraneous noise in the room. Listen for:

- *Audience noises*-Coughs, sidebar conversations, shuffling feet, etc.

- *Environmental noises:* Heat or air conditioning blowers, voices outside the door or windows, and noises from equipment like projectors or VCRs.

- *Speaker noises:* Hands that tap the lectern, jewelry rattling, fabrics rustling, or feet shuffling.

Although these distractions may be obvious to you, it's quite possible that the speaker is not even aware of the noises. Assume you are now the speaker and consider these questions:

1. What techniques can you use to alert yourself to the noises? _____

    _____

    _____

2. How would you adapt to or eliminate these distractions?

    _____

    _____

    _____

3. Is there anything you can do in advance of the speech to eliminate the noise? _____

    _____

    _____

Note: You should know the name of the maintenance person in charge of your room in case you need to contact her before or during your presentation. You might also want to have a "plant" in the audience who can alert you to any problems.

Chapter 11

Using Notes That Work for You

Good speaker notes can be a lifesaver. Bad notes . . . well, let's not think about them. Most speakers use notes of some kind. Even professional presenters who appear to have no notes often have teleprompters or cue cards. Politicians, stand-up comedians, and talk show hosts have help sounding spontaneous. Speaking without notes is like walking the tightrope without a net—unpredictable and dangerous!

Use notes because notes:

- Keep you focused on your structure. Think of them as a road map. Notes can reduce the tendency to stray from your goal and can assist in getting you easily from your starting point to your destination.
- Get you back on track if your train of thought derails and you "go blank." You can go directly to the next point on your note card and get right back on the road to your destination.
- Provide an excellent security blanket and give added confidence to a nervous speaker. Well-prepared notes can help a speaker sound self-assured and natural.

Preparing Your Notes

If you take a public speaking class, most professors give instructions on the kind of note cards they expect students to use. If you receive a grade on your note cards, *construct them exactly as instructed by your professor*! If you are speaking outside an academic setting, you have plenty of freedom to choose a style of note preparation that works for you. Use the tips presented here within the restrictions dictated by your instructor or your corporate culture.

USE CARDS FOR PRESENTATIONS UNDER 15 MINUTES.

Standard 3×5-inch note cards are less conspicuous than a sheet of paper. If your hands have a tendency to shake, it is less noticeable to the audience when you carry smaller note cards. Cards don't rustle or make as much noise as larger, thinner sheets of paper when you move them.

There are, however, some exceptions to the note card rule. Presentations of over 15 minutes require so many notes that cards become cumbersome. Standard 8½×11-inch paper is your best choice for long presentations. Some speakers simply prefer notes typed on the computer because they're neater and can be stored in memory. If you choose to type your notes, use a large font

(18 point minimum)

to ensure good visibility. If you use handwritten notes, print large and legibly.

Hint: If you are giving your presentation more than once or if you might later need to remember all the specifics of what you have said, make sure to type or scan your notes into a computer. You can easily misplace your notes between speaking engagements. The computer provides a backup so that you won't permanently lose them. Another key benefit to the computer is that you can save different versions of the notes. This way, you can adapt the presentation without a total rewrite. You can go back and review the different versions to remember exactly what you said to each group.

USE KEY WORDS.

Don't write out the speech on your cards. Use key words to focus on the points you want to make. Key words allow you to talk your way through the speech, sounding fresh and natural as you speak. There are, of course, a few exceptions:

- Write out quotes to ensure accuracy.

- Write out statistics as well as the specific statements you'll make if you rephrase the numbers to make them more easily understood.

- Write out any information requiring specific detail.

- Use a script when dealing with highly sensitive information. When there is no room for misinterpretation, read from the script.

- Many speakers write out introductions and conclusions and state them verbatim.

INCLUDE TRANSITIONAL PHRASES IN YOUR NOTES.

This ensures that you move smoothly from point to point. Again, don't write out the full sentence, just a phrase or two to help you remember the appropriate way to make the transition.

USE ONE SIDE ONLY.

Print notes on only one side of the card or sheet of paper. Flipping cards over can distract the audience and confuse the speaker.

NUMBER YOUR NOTE CARDS.

Number each page boldly in the upper right-hand corner. This is a good preventative measure. In case cards are dropped or mixed up, you can get them back in numerical order. Don't staple or bind your notes. Loose notes can be turned like pages of a book.

USE AS FEW CARDS AS POSSIBLE.

The more cards you have, the more potential there is for confusion and distraction. You might be tempted to write out information in great detail, "just in case" you forget something. *Don't talk yourself into doing this!* When you stand before an audience, the written word can act like a magnet and your eyes will irresistibly go to the cards. This eliminates any chance for you to look or sound natural. Fewer cards can help the verbal and visual flow to stay smooth. After you give a few presentations, you quickly learn how many cards, containing how much information, work for you. This number varies from person to person.

WRITE STAGE DIRECTIONS ON YOUR NOTES.

Remember that no one sees your notes but you. It's perfectly acceptable to mark up the notes any way you please. Just make sure you know what your marks mean. The simpler your system, the better. If you plan to ask a question, turn to a flip chart, or hold up a prop, mark your instructions on the left side of your notes.

USE COLOR.

Use the same color scheme for your cards each time you prepare a speech. The colors you use are a matter of personal preference, but remember that certain colors are far easier to see than others. For instance, yellow is an excellent highlight color, but does not work well for text. A simple technique for handwritten notes is to use blue for text and red for stage instructions in the left margin and black for any last minute additions to the speech.

BRING AN EXTRA COPY.

Make a photocopy of your notes and keep it with you the day of your speech. Put it in a back pocket, a backpack, briefcase, or even your shoe if you choose! Just keep it somewhere other than where you keep the first version. Think of the extra copy like a "just-in-case-you-get-locked-out-key" that you may have for your home or car. This technique has saved several students from having to "wing it" without notes.

Practicing with Your Cards

PRACTICE WITH THE REAL NOTES.

Some speakers use "practice" notes for practicing their speech, then make a clean copy for the actual presentation. This is not a good idea because we become familiar with the old notes. It's preferable to use the same copy of your notes for practicing that you'll use for the real presentation. You'll get used to the spacing and design of your cards and be comfortable with any handwritten notes or pictures you may have drawn on the cards. All these little things help retention and contribute to a better final presentation.

RECREATE THE REAL SITUATION.

Practice in an environment like that of the actual presentation. This may even mean creating your own lectern to place the notes on. This can be done with cardboard boxes or books. Try to create the same height and width of the lectern or table you will use. If you need to hold your cards in the formal presentation, it's important to practice while holding them. This lets you feel comfortable with your gestures and practice your eye contact. Practice as often as you can in a room the size of the one where you'll formally present.

KEEP NOTES INCONSPICUOUS.

Practice before the video camera to check yourself for the way you turn or move your cards or papers. Notes should be as unobtrusive as possible, supporting your speech, not detracting from it.

Using Cards during the Presentation

CARRY YOUR CARDS IN ONE HAND.

Carry your notes with you as you approach the lectern. Carrying note cards in a coat pocket can cause an embarrassing situation. It's easy to drop cards while taking them out of a pocket, and playing "52 pickup" is a terrible way to begin a speech. Simply carrying your cards inconspicuously in one hand is usually the best and safest technique. If you use typed sheets, carry them in a simple folder with pockets.

DO NOT HOLD NOTE CARDS.

Whenever possible, place your cards on a lectern or a small side table. This keeps your cards from drawing attention and hides the nervous hand shaking, if any. Do not under any circumstances *hold* a full-sized sheet while speaking. It's guaranteed to distract the audience and the barrier to gestures annoys the speaker.

LOOK AT YOUR AUDIENCE, NOT YOUR NOTES.

For some inexperienced speakers, the note cards become a security blanket. The speaker's eyes stay on the notes, but they don't *see* anything. Try to look at the notes only when it's time to move to a new point or when you truly need to see what comes next.

DON'T MEMORIZE.

A goal of most presenters is to sound as natural as possible. Most of us don't sound the least bit natural when we recite a memorized script. Even some actors have a difficult time sounding natural when they're trying to be themselves. Public speaking calls on a different set of skills than acting. A primary difference is that you do not play a character. You are yourself up there. Be the *best you* that you can be. Be the "you" who stands up straight, uses good grammar, is confident and charming. By the time you give your presentation, you will have practiced enough that you'll know each point that you want to make. The the way you say it should come naturally.

DON'T REARRANGE NOTE CARDS.

When you finish the information on one note card and are ready to go on to the next, move the used card from right to left on the lectern. Do not turn the card over or place it behind the other cards, simply move it out of the way and go on to the next card. You can put the cards back in order after your presentation.

Using notes will help you feel more comfortable and can make you look more professional.

Sample Note Card

Part Two
Three sales mediums   (blue)
  Benefits—
    fastest response
    significant results

(Turn to flip chart)   (red)

Methods   (blue)
 • Direct Sales by existing organizations
     Representatives of other
       organizations will sell the product
       for us   (blue)

 • Telemarketing   (blue)
     Rob will address our plan.   (black)
     Market direct to the consumer   (blue)

 • Direct Sales by B2 Inc.   (blue)
     Principals of B2 will sell direct to
       corporations or non-profit groups

Chapter 12

Visual Aids

Good visual aids add credibility to your presentation and keep the attention of the audience. What you show an audience has about three times as much impact as what you tell them.

Example

Think of the Vietnam War. What have you been told and what do you remember? What mental images come to mind? Chances are you think of images of young soldiers fighting in the jungle and protesters in the United States. Almost everyone who participates in this exercise quickly remembers a picture embedded in their brain of a young girl running down a street crying in pain, her naked body burned by napalm.

One picture . . . a thousand words.

Visual aids consist of anything used to support your message. You need to know the various kinds of visual aids, know how to prepare them, and know the best ways to use them.

Kinds of Visual Aids

OBJECTS

Using objects in a presentation can clarify or emphasize your points. This might be the real object you're discussing or something representing a concept.

Example

For a simple science demonstration on the solar system, a basketball could be used to represent the sun, a tennis ball for the earth, and a marble might be the moon.

MODELS

Sometimes the real item is too large, too small, or too cumbersome to actually show during your presentation.

Example

Bringing a car engine or a motorcycle into a meeting room or most classrooms would not be appropriate. A model or a depiction of the actual item would be a good representation.

THE SPEAKER

Sometimes the speaker can act as a visual aid himself.

Example

A speech on healthy lifestyles and getting into shape can be illustrated by the speaker actually demonstrating exercises. This is very effective if the speaker dresses appropriately and looks in shape! If the speaker is someone who simply *wants* to get in shape, he has no credibility with the audience.

PHOTOGRAPHS AND POSTERS

An enlarged photograph can work in helping the audience visualize exactly what you describe.

Example

If you speak about San Francisco, set the tone with posters of the Golden Gate Bridge and the city skyline.

SLIDES

Slide projections are large and, if well prepared, are easy to read and visually very pleasing. The major drawback to using slides is that the room must be darkened and the speaker is invisible. The entire presentation *becomes* the slide. Slides can also be misplaced; so bring a backup set if possible. Practice without your slides at least once, just in case.

TRANSPARENCIES

Unlike slides, transparencies can be used in normal room lighting. Transparencies are inexpensive, easy to produce, and user-friendly. You can convert most graphs, drawings, and pictures to transparency slides. Color can be an important part of the presentation. Color is introduced by using a color printer with specially designed transparency film or by making color copies on appropriate transparency film. You can also convert pictures produced on a color copier to transparencies.

VIDEOS

Supplementing a presentation with a well chosen, carefully edited video segment can work effectively. A presentation about "All-Time Great Stars of the NBA" can have much more impact with quick clips of the best shots of Dr. J, Michael Jordan, and Kareem Abdoul Jabar interspersed.

A drawback to using videos is that VCRs are getting more complicated and "technical difficulties" have caused many embarrassing moments. Prepare a backup way to give your presentation without the support of a video, just in case.

FLIP CHART SHEETS

There are several advantages to using a flip chart:

- You can prepare pages in advance.
- You can move the whole flip chart to a better spot in the room at any time.
- You can tear pages off and post them all around the room.

The flip chart can also be very interactive. The presenter or an appointed scribe can write lists as the audience calls out answers to your questions. Use wide, bright markers to write on the pages of the flip chart. Use masking tape as tabs to make turning pages easier.

Note: Do not use a flip chart in a large room or with over 50 people in the audience. The larger format of transparencies works better in larger settings.

COMPUTER-GENERATED GRAPHICS

Many software packages produce beautiful graphics. Most "works" packages produced by major software companies can easily create a multitude of pictures and graphics. Several other software programs help speakers prepare speaker notes and excellent visual aids. Many business schools and companies use the PowerPoint program, which produces professional graphics in an easy-to-learn format.

Warning: These programs make it easy to use wordy graphics for everything you'll say. Remember that visual aids are intended to be "visual." Don't be seduced into creating an outline as your visual aid. When in doubt whether a written word or picture would best support your point, choose the picture.

Computers and software are not foolproof. A nervous presenter and an unfamiliar computer can be a dangerous combination. Even the most experienced speaker can have a disaster with a malfunctioning computer-generated program. Always bring hardcopy or transparency backups.

When a bulb burns out, the computer freezes up, or a video tape tears and won't play, take no more than five minutes to attempt repairs. Any more time tends to alienate your audience as you ignore them while you work with equipment. Go to your backup plan after five minutes and begin your presentation. A less than perfect presentation is better than a thirty-minute delay.

Preparing Visual Aids

PREPARE IN ADVANCE.

Any visual aid should support your presentation, not distract from it. The speaker therefore needs to ensure that it looks right and functions correctly. Check and double check each chart, transparency, prop, and object you plan to use. Make sure there are no typos and that each supporting item you use actually does what it is intended to do. Many presentations have been damaged by last-minute decisions to add visual aids.

MAKE SURE THAT VISUALS ARE JUST THAT—VISUAL.

Don't crowd a slide with the full outline of what you will say. Words are one of the least effective things you can put on a slide. Use pictures, graphs, drawings, or models, with words simply supplementing the visual, not dominating them. Remember that *visual* aids are designed to support your speech, not outline it. When you choose to put words on your graphics, remember that the audience gives a lot of credit to the printed word: Make the words important ones.

KEEP IT SIMPLE.

- Use clean and uncluttered visual aids. Complex slides or props serve more to distract the audience than help them.
- Use only one chart or graph per slide.
- Supplement only one concept or idea per slide.
- Use only one font per slide whenever possible. If it helps to get your point across, you can use two fonts, but *never* use more than two.

USE BULLET POINTS.

Do not print text with long phrases on a slide. Use short phrases in a bullet point form. Never use full sentences for text unless you display an exact quote. Some organizational cultures almost require that slides contain words. If you face this situation, as a general rule, a slide should not contain more than five lines and no more than six words per line.

USE LARGE PRINT.

Your entire audience needs to see your visual aid clearly and easily. Keep it large and bold. Print should be readable to the naked eye at a distance of 10 feet. The minimum type to use on a transparency should be 24 point and looks like this:

24-point type

Larger type is often better.

MAKE IT MEANINGFUL.

If a visual aid is not necessary to support something you are saying, don't use it. Make sure it clarifies, makes your message more meaningful, or immortalizes it. For example, most statistics are easier to understand when supported with an illustration, photographs of people help the audience identify with them, and a cartoon can make a point for you. Don't be caught up in the trend of using a visual aid for each point you make.

USE COLOR TO KEEP VISUALS ALIVE.

Use four or fewer colors per slide. When using graphs, be consistent in using a specific color to represent a specific item.

Tips for Using Support Materials

PRACTICE, PRACTICE, PRACTICE.

To ensure that each prop works and your presentation flows smoothly, you must practice using the prop exactly as you'll use it in your actual speech. When things go wrong, a speaker can look quite foolish. You want your audience to remember your presentation for its top quality, not for its comedy value.

DON'T READ.

Your task is public speaking, not public reading! Watching a speaker read the entire presentation from slides is boring and distracting to the audience. In fact, there is no need for a speaker if the entire content can be read.

TALK TO THE AUDIENCE, NOT TO THE PROP.

Most of us have seen a speaker have a conversation with a slide or prop while standing in front of an audience. In the long run, the speaker ends up looking foolish and the audience becomes annoyed. Turn to face the audience as you speak. Your eyes should be face front and should remain on the audience about 85% of the time.

TIME YOUR VISUAL AIDS.

Your visual aid is for the benefit of your audience. Be aware of the length of time you expose the visual aid. In general, show a model or slide for at least 30 seconds so that the audience has time to view and comprehend what you're showing them. In most instances, you should show your visual aid for no more than two minutes. Do not leave a slide on when you have finished talking about it. If you won't be using a slide for a minute or more, simply turn off the projector. *Never* offend the eyeballs of your audience by leaving a projector on without a transparency.

KEEP A CLEAR VIEW.

Be conscious of how you stand when using slides or transparencies. Be aware of the line of sight of the people to your left and right. If you must stand in front of them for part of the time, be sure to move so that everyone can see most of the time.

Make sure that your shoulder on your writing side is not in the projected view. Check this by looking at your shoulder while holding your body perfectly still. If the light projects onto your shoulder, you are blocking the view.

Keep the screen at the front of the room, high enough for those at the back of the room to see clearly. As a rule of thumb, the bottom of the screen should be at least 48 inches from the floor. If you cannot control the placement of the screen, adjust the projector so that you use only the recommended portion of the screen. If possible, place the projector to the right of a right-handed speaker and to the left of a left-handed speaker. That placement makes gesturing more natural and allows for the speaker to write on a transparency without blocking the view.

KEEP EXTRA COPIES.

For every transparency and slide, keep an extra copy with you at the front of the room. This serves two purposes. First, in case your slides get lost, you have extra copies and you don't look foolish saying, "Well, now I would have been showing you a graph of . . . ." You can also use a paper copy of your transparencies for notes as you speak. This keeps you from looking at the projected slide and keeps your eyes facing front.

THINK BEFORE PASSING ITEMS AROUND THE AUDIENCE.

When you pass things among a group of people, their attention is automatically drawn to the item and away from the speaker. If you have an important point to make, you may choose to simply hold the item up for all to see or wait until you have finished speaking to pass it around. The same applies to any handouts you may use. If you pass out an outline of your presentation, you can bet the audience will read ahead and reach the end of your speech before you do.

EXPLAIN ANY VISUAL YOU USE.

Don't use a visual that you don't reference. The audience will wonder what the visual means or may simply be distracted by it. If you don't need it, don't use it. If you use it, explain it!

Try your skill with visual aids in the following exercises.

Exercises

MAKING APPROPRIATE CHOICES

Objective

To choose appropriate visual aids for different speech topics.

Method

For each of the following topics, list three visual aids that you feel would best support the main message.

1. How snakes adjust to seasonal changes

_____

_____

_____

2. Small talk and the art of mingling

_____

_____

_____

3. Why cigarette vending machines must be outlawed

_____

_____

_____

4. The comedy of Jerry Seinfeld

_____

_____

_____

5. Why to invest in the U.S. stock market *today*

_____

_____

_____

6. How to juggle

_____

_____

_____

7. Writing for television

_____

_____

_____

8. The Siberian tiger

_____

_____

_____

9. How not to give a speech

_____

_____

_____

10. The most successful marketing campaigns of Pepsi Cola

_____

_____

_____

The answers are on the following page.

1. How snakes adjust to seasonal changes
   a. *Not* a real snake unless you let the audience know ahead of time, so that any squeamish listeners can leave the room or move to the back
   b. Pictures of snakes before and after they shed their skin
   c. Poster with a chart listing behavioral changes at differing temperatures
2. Small talk and the art of mingling
   a. Pictures of people in conversation
   b. Volunteers from the audience to role-play scenarios you have created
   c. Transparency with five successful "opening lines" for meeting someone
3. Why cigarette machines must be outlawed
   a. Slides of very young children smoking cigarettes
   b. Change to equal the cost of a pack of cigarettes and a jar stained with brown wood stain. You can make the statement that, "This is all it costs to turn clean lungs into lungs that look like this jar."
   c. Graph of total vending machine sales of tobacco products
4. The comedy of Jerry Seinfeld
   a. Short video clips of Seinfeld's best performances
   b. Poster from a recent live performance
   c. Transparency image, "Did you ever notice . . .?"
5. Why to invest in the U.S. stock market *today*
   a. Graph of Nasdaq performance over the last ten years compared to bank savings accounts
   b. Play money to equal the value of both figures on the previous graph
   c. Poster showing the financial concept of "the power of 72"

6. How to juggle
   a. Juggling balls
   b. Volunteers to teach
   c. Handout of the steps to follow to learn simple juggling
7. Writing for television
   a. Actual TV script
   b. Handout comparison of well-written page and a poorly written page
   c. A remote control to symbolize what the audience does to a poorly written show
8. The Siberian tiger
   a. Poster of tigers
   b. Plaster mold of tiger teeth
   c. Video of tiger attacking prey
9. How not to give a speech [This is an excellent opportunity to go for the laugh and make the speech your own comedy routine.]
   a. The speaker can be a visual aid, acting out humorous scenes
   b. A very long computer printout to be used as an example of having too many notes
   c. Examples of posters with small print and poor graphics
10. The most successful marketing campaigns of Pepsi Cola
   a. Samples of Pepsi products
   b. Pictures of Pepsi ads through the last century
   c. Pepsi T-shirts, key chains, bumper stickers, etc.

USES ON TELEVISION

Objectives

To observe and be consciously aware of the use of visual aids on television.

To determine which visual aids work well in specific situations.

Method

Watch several news programs within a one- to two-day period. Observe how graphics and models are used to support the message. Observe which programs use the same graphic for the same news story. Try turning away from the television and listening to the story. Turn back and watch the screen. Does the graphic make the information clearer? Does it add or detract from the message? Does it appear that the story was written "around" the graphic?

Ask yourself whether the supporting material does any of these things:

- Maintain attention?
- Supplement the message?
- Prove a point?
- Add variety to the presentation?
- Give lasting impact to the story?

Note: Do not assume that all news programs use visual aids appropriately or that you should model your presentations after them.

Chapter 13

Keeping Them Tuned In

The average attention span of an adult is not much longer than that of a child. We tend to mentally "tune in and out" while we're listening. We mentally alter our attention from what the speaker is saying to other things we could be doing, what we would like to have for lunch, and how to choose a name for our new puppy before we return to the speaker's message. Consequently, speakers not only have to *get* the attention of the audience, they have to keep *regaining* it!

This chapter shows you ways to maintain an audience's interest.

Using the Voice

The speaker's voice should sound natural, yet controlled and professional. The actress Fran Dresher, who played TV's "The Nanny," has become famous for her natural voice. Each sound is drawn out in a nasal whine that delights many listeners and sends others rushing for the remote! Most speakers would *not* choose this speaking style.

Listen to yourself on audio or video tape. Consider the following vocal qualities when you determine ways to keep the audience tuned in.

PITCH

This is the high or low musical quality of your voice. Is your voice more like a tuba (a bass) or a flute (a soprano)? Use your natural pitch for best results.

RANGE

The group of notes from low to high that your voice reaches comfortably and naturally is your range. The more notes you're comfortable using, the more variety your speaking voice has. Use a wide range to avoid a monotone.

VOLUME

Volume is the loudness and force you use to project your voice. A booming voice can make the audience sit back in their seats. Too much volume can be intimidating and offensive. A more common problem is when a speaker uses too little volume. If you make the audience *work* to hear what you have to say, they won't listen long. They may judge you as lacking confidence or competence.

Make sure to project from the diaphragm. The diaphragm is a muscle just below the rib cage. Singers and musicians who play brass or wind instruments must breathe from the diaphragm to sustain the quality of notes they play. Practice this type of breathing regularly. Exhale breaths that are longer and deeper than normal. Feel as if you're squeezing a toothpaste tube from the bottom rather than the middle.

Tip: A loud voice *often* gets the attention of your audience. A long pause followed by quietly spoken words *always* gets their attention. Silence is your most powerful tool. If you find your audience is visibly bored or begins to chat with each other while you're on stage, try ten seconds of silence. This normally gets everyone's attention. Change your position on stage, lower your voice, and use direct eye contact with the audience. Insert some humor and involve the audience by asking them to do something or answer questions. This should get them back. (See Chapter 14 "What You Don't Say Speaks Louder than Words," for more techniques.)

RATE

The pace, quickness, and tempo of your speech pattern determine the rate. Vary your rate of speech during a presentation to keep attention. Don't race to the end and don't plod along.

Most listeners prefer to hear a moderately fast, resonant voice. Changing your resonance takes a lot of work. But it's not hard to speak reasonably quickly and loudly. If you find you have persistent problems with any of these qualities, ask a teacher or speech coach for a little individual attention. There are simple exercises that can improve almost any problem.

Using Language

ENUNCIATION

The way you make the distinct sounds within a word is important for your audience to understand your message. Sound out words crisply. Don't slur together sounds like "gonna" in place of "going to" or "'sup?" instead of "What's up?"

PRONUNCIATION

Say words in the way the dictionary suggests.

Examples
In grade school, most of us were taught to say library instead of "liberry".

Other common problems include:
"I axed you" instead of "I asked you."
"Expresso" coffee instead of "espresso."
"Excape" instead of "escape."

When in doubt, look it up. Even if your family members say a word one way, they aren't necessarily right!

DENOTATION AND CONNOTATION

Denotation is the dictionary meaning of the word. *Connotation* is the meaning gained through society's accepted definition of a word.

Example
Take the word *cool.* Prior to the 1960s, *cool* meant a chilly temperature, aloof, or calm. Today, *cool* means those things as well as something good or interesting.

A *blast* means an explosion, storm or reprimand, but when used to describe a party, it means a good time.

There are cultural differences in the denotation of words. Be cautious if your audience doesn't know you. If you are uncomfortable with the meaning of any words or phrases, check with a trusted friend who knows the culture of the audience.

SIMILE AND METAPHOR

These techniques compare one thing to another. A speaker uses *simile* when he says one thing is "like" another. Simile involves the words "like" or "as."

Examples
A new yellow car might be described as "bright as day."

When something happens suddenly, it's "like a bolt of lightning."

Metaphor makes a comparison directly, calling one thing something else.

Examples
His eyes danced.

She thundered through the room.

These techniques add interest to your message.

VISUAL WORDS

Use words that create a visual picture in the audience's mind.

Example
To describe a thunderstorm, you could say, "The sky was dark and it was raining hard." You might better say, "The clouds rolled as the sky turned from blue to gray and from gray to charcoal. Rain poured like streams from buckets."

When the audience can visualize your words, they can embody them.

SIMPLE WORDS

Make the complex as simple as possible. If you must share detailed information, state the facts as simply as possible and follow your description with a handout listing all appropriate information.

REPETITION

Repeat key words and rephrase important points intermittently to help the audience remember your message. State statistics in several ways to make them understandable and memorable.

STREAMLINE

Don't overload your presentation with too much material. Divide a long, information-loaded presentation into shorter, more comprehensible segments. Audiences can't retain huge amounts of information in one sitting. Supplement verbal information with visual aids and written handouts to aid retention.

EAR-FRIENDLY LANGUAGE

Choose and structure words that sound natural. In most situations, you should sound conversational, but not casual. Sentence structure that is acceptable in print may be ineffective when spoken aloud.

Example

A newspaper article may read, "'The council members are frustrated with the new voting procedure,' the mayor said."

This is obviously unacceptable in a speech. Instead, you could say, "The mayor announced that the council members are frustrated with the new voting process."

To keep your audience tuned in, use your voice and language carefully. (See Chapter 14, "What You Don't Say Speaks Louder than Words," for nonverbal techniques to keep attention.)

Try the following exercises to keep your audience tuned in.

Exercises

THE SOUND OF YOUR VOICE

Objective

To become familiar with the sound of your own voice

Materials

Use an audio tape recorder.

Method

Record yourself reading a children's story or a newspaper. You'll need only 5 to 10 minutes of taped material. Enlist the help of a friend or business professional to act as your coach. Listen to your pitch, range, volume, and rate. Does the sound of your voice send the message you want to send about yourself?

Listen to the way you pronounce and enunciate words. Ask your coach if you are accurate. Do you speak clearly and understandably? If you discover specific problem areas, practice reading to improve the problem. If working alone doesn't help, call a local university to find a voice and articulation coach. Most problems can be corrected.

EAR-FRIENDLY LANGUAGE

Objectives

To become aware of language that sounds natural when spoken aloud.

To learn to choose ear-friendly words for presentations.

Materials

The tools for this exercise include newspapers, magazines, and professionally prepared radio or television copy. An audio or video camera is useful but not necessary for this exercise.

Method

This can be done individually or in a group. Read a newspaper aloud and listen to how awkward some phrases sound. Speaking style is different from good writing style. It is more conversational and flows easily off the tongue. Compare newspaper writing to prepared radio or television copy. Watch a broadcaster or listen to radio news to check for differences.

Chapter 14

What You Don't Say Speaks Louder than Words

Verbal communication includes the words that we say. Nonverbal communication involves *how* we communicate what we have to say.

Nonverbal communication takes place constantly. Each sigh, yawn, smile, and raise of the eyebrow says something. A frequently used phrase is, "We cannot *not* communicate nonverbally."

Elements of Nonverbal Communication

DISTANCES

How close or far we stand from someone tells them something about us. We can make them comfortable or feel we are uncomfortable and quite formal just by adjusting our distance and space. The way we organize our office or dorm room sets a tone.

In his classic 1969 book, *The Hidden Dimension,* Edward Hall defined four distances that Americans observe without consciously being aware.

Intimate	Touch–18 inches
Personal	18 inches–4 feet
Social	4 feet–12 feet
Public	12 feet or more

Our comfort level varies according to who enters each of these zones. When a stranger enters our personal or intimate zones, we usually back up to establish a more comfortable distance.

Example

This tendency was demonstrated on the popular sitcom "Seinfeld" in a classic episode featuring the "close talker." In this episode, Elaine's boyfriend stands just inches from the other person when he speaks, causing all the other cast members to slowly move away until each has been backed against a wall.

Use this technique to your advantage if you're speaking to a small or medium-sized group. If two or more members of your audience are having a private conversation while you're speaking, keep talking while walking toward them. Do not look at them, simply approach and stand near them while you continue with what you were saying. Their conversation normally stops and you do not embarrass them or break the pace of your presentation.

Classroom and conference room presentations usually take place in the social distance. Normally, any situation that involves speaking before a group larger than 25 or addressing any size group from a stage, takes place in the public distance.

THE SOUND OF OUR VOICE

The tone (pitch or quality), volume (loudness), and rate (speed) we use to speak all contribute to communication. Many vocal factors affect how we communicate. (See Chapter 13, "Keeping Them Tuned In," for more information.)

POSTURE

Simply standing straight or in a slumped way sends a strong positive or negative message to anyone watching you. To appear positive and confident, choose the "centered position" in which you distribute your weight evenly on both feet and hold your arms comfortably at your sides. If you serve as a panel member or if you sit at the head table waiting for an introduction, look alert and sit up straight.

Remember that you are "on stage" at all times and your audience judges you *before* you even speak.

FACIAL EXPRESSIONS

We can easily identify the difference between a smile, a scowl, a wink, and a blank stare. Just as easily, we attach meanings to those expressions. Expressions like a grimace, a knitted eyebrow, or a grin can add more meaning to our words. A speaker should make sure that facial expressions and the intended meaning behind the words match. Sometimes a nervous speaker smiles without being aware of it. This sends a poor message when the topic is serious. Just as often, nerves keep some speakers from demonstrating any facial expression at all. An audience can't get excited about a topic that doesn't appear to excite the speaker. When you practice with the video camera, check for appropriate facial expressions during all parts of your presentation.

Example
You say, "The book was really good," but you roll your eyes and speak sarcastically. The audience believes the nonverbal behavior over the spoken words.

EYE CONTACT

In the culture of the United States, direct eye contact indicates trustworthiness, friendliness, and confidence. Averted eyes usually indicate just the opposite. Ask yourself this question: Would you prefer to have a conversation with someone who looks at you most of the time or someone who looks at her shoes, the ceiling, or someone else? Most of us prefer to speak with someone looking at us. The audience prefers good eye contact too. If you are particularly nervous about looking people in the eye while you're speaking and you have the opportunity to speak before a large audience of 25 or more, look them in the forehead! Find a spot just above the nose and at a distance of over 10 feet it looks as though you're looking them in the eyes!

Averted eyes don't communicate confidence, but neither does staring behavior. When a speaker stares at the deci-

sion maker, she excludes the rest of the audience and probably makes the decision maker uncomfortable.

GESTURES

How we use our hands can speak volumes.

Example
In most places in the United States, a wave of the hand means hello
or good-bye.

In Hawaii, the little finger and thumb indicate "hang loose."

Maybe you remember seeing your mom put her hands on her hips
just before telling you something you did wrong. The position of her
hands alone let you know that what she would say was not good
news.

In a presentation, gestures can show any number of
emotions and express a variety of sentiments.

Examples
A pointed finger or crossed arms may signal hostility.

Finger tapping on the lectern telegraphs anxiety.

Continually touching the face could mean embarrassment or insin-
cerity.

Use natural gestures and control them.

Examples
Use a two-handed, open palm movement to emphasize a point, but
do not let your arms flail uncontrollably or too frequently.

Unlike facial expressions, gestures are culturally bound.

Example
The peace sign or "OK" symbol might indicate something perverse
in another culture.

BODY MOVEMENT

Use movement purposefully. An inexperienced speaker
sometimes has so much adrenaline running through his
body that he begins to "dance" behind the lectern. The
speaker may not notice that she continually shifts her
weight from her right foot to her left while speaking. The
audience watching the dance notices, however, and may feel

a little seasick! Try to find a balance between too little and too much movement. Standing stiff and totally motionless can be as detrimental to imparting a message as pacing uncontrollably. If you pace, the audience watches your pacing and ignores what you say.

Here are some hints to combat uncontrollable movements:

- As you walk to the front of the room to begin your speech, find the spot where you will stand to start your presentation.

- Plant your feet solidly on the floor. Men should stand in the "ready position" with feet a shoulder width apart, knees slightly bent. Women can assume the same stance or if they prefer a slightly more feminine stance, try a modified ready position with feet about six inches apart, one foot facing forward and one foot at about a 30-degree angle.

- Once you are "planted" at the front of the room, keep your feet in the same position for at least 30 seconds before choosing to move. If you choose to move to a new position, take at least two steps and "plant" your feet again. Stay in that position for at least 30 seconds before moving again. The 30-second minimum rule keeps a speaker from appearing to pace. A polished speaker will time her movements to indicate transitions from one point of the speech to the next. This adds emphasis and nonverbally signals the audience that a new point is coming.

All of these elements of nonverbal communication add up to our general appearance. To be a good speaker, the content of your presentation *must* be good. How you sound and look can help or hurt your credibility as a speaker.

We don't always know how we look to others. We must rely on pictures, mirrors, the comments of others, and video tape to get an idea. Has anyone ever asked you something like why you were mad or what was so funny? You probably hadn't said anything, but somehow they perceived that you were mad or silently laughing. That's nonverbal communication in action.

When verbal and nonverbal cues don't match, the nonverbal cues usually provide a key to the true meaning of the message.

Example

An acquaintance says, "I'm really glad to see you" and is looking over your shoulder at someone else. Do you believe him?

A good presentation requires that verbal and nonverbal communication match.

Determining Your Nonverbal Cues

Video tape yourself to test your own nonverbal messages. Then review the tape with a friend who acts as a speech coach. Watch the tape at least *three times*. If you're not used to seeing yourself on tape, during the first viewing you criticize everything you see. The second viewing is more realistic. Finally, the third time through, you start to see that you also did many positive things!

When you watch the tape, keep three things in mind:

1. Your voice really does sound like that.
2. Your hair really does look like that.
3. You are *not* that heavy! The camera adds 10 to 15 pounds to all of us.

Nonwords

In addition to listening to the words you speak, listen to the other sounds you make. Most inexperienced speakers should pay particular attention to the nonwords like "um," "ah," and "and." Many of us fall into patterns when we use these sounds. Some people fill the pauses between sentences or words with an "uhhh," often uttered in a long drawn-out single tone. This almost sounds like singing and doesn't allow a break in the monologue. Other people use

144

nonwords in a short stacatto style in the beginning or middle of a sentence.

Look out for the favorite phrases "like" and "you know." These common fillers for the Generation X age group are acceptable in normal conversation among peers, but not in presentations. People from previous generations find those fillers annoying and distracting.

Along with common age-specific language, certain regions also have their own idiosyncratic patterns of speech.

Example

In central Illinois, the people who put groceries in bags for shoppers to take home are called "sackers."

In western Pennsylvania, when a person cleans up his home before company comes to visit, he is said to "red up" the house.

Most of us know the southern phrase "y'all."

Be aware of your regional speaking habits since people from other areas may consider terms common to you to be nonwords.

Some of us get into the habit of frequently repeating one phrase or word unconsciously like "actually," "basically," and "you see." Listen for this pattern while you watch yourself on tape. If a speaker has this habit, the audience stops hearing the presentation and starts counting the repeated phrase.

After you and your coach discuss your performance, go back and rework the wording and concentrate on improving any nonverbal language that didn't please you. Make sure you do at least one more taped performance, practicing your "new and improved" style. It's important for you to see that you look and sound better. It's almost a guarantee that you improve between the first and second tapings—if you make the effort!

How others perceive you is critical in your interaction. Perception may not be accurate, but to the perceiver it is reality! Your first impression may color your relationship with this individual for months to come.

Top Ten Negative Nonverbal Cues (Before, During, and After Your Presentation)

WEAK HANDSHAKE

Both men and women in the American culture shake hands frequently. The "limp" handshake from either gender is perceived poorly. The web between the thumb and forefinger should touch the web of the other person's hand and the "squeeze" should be firm but not hard. Men in business settings should not give women the fingers-only grip. Even if the intent is to be polite, the message can be demeaning. Watch for anyone who has an obvious injury or an older person with swollen knuckles. If someone has hand pain, you do not want to make it worse. A gentle, polite handshake works well.

SLOPPY CLOTHES

Treat your presentation like a job interview. Wear something that makes you look good, is moderately conservative, and fits well. Choose something appropriate for the setting and the audience. If you present before a group wearing "business casual" clothes, you may choose not to wear a suit; your own *best* business casual may be appropriate. Make sure everything is clean and freshly pressed. Double check your shoes for worn spots or the need for polish. In the classroom, dress a cut above the way you normally dress. Generally, we behave more professionally when we're dressed more professionally; so give yourself the edge with your attire.

TOO MUCH JEWELRY

Wear conservative jewelry for your presentation. Large or flashy pieces distract your audience. Jewelry that doesn't move too much is the best choice. Earrings shouldn't dangle and bracelets shouldn't jingle. Men who wear earrings should consider whether the audience will accept your jewelry.

INAPPROPRIATE HAIRSTYLE

Choose a stylish hairstyle, not a trendy one, as well as something appropriate for your age and career or student status. If you've ever seen a make-over on TV or in a magazine, you can see what a big difference a new hairstyle can make. When you look in the mirror and see someone from the last decade, it's time for a change.

SLOUCHING

Whether you're sitting or standing, keep your back straight and your shoulders back. Simply making this one change makes you look and sound more confident. Slouching implies apathy whether you sit or stand.

STARING AT YOUR NOTES

Looking directly at an audience helps them connect with you as a person. Most American audiences have more trust and confidence in people who look directly at them. Those who keep their eyes on notes or a visual aid disconnect themselves from the audience and lose the advantage of feedback.

BAD BREATH

When you are speaking one on one, bad breath can be alienating. When it's important to make a positive impression, keep a few mints handy so that you don't have to worry about this problem. Don't chew gum or eat mints while giving your presentation.

DIRTY FINGERNAILS

This is easily corrected. Double check your hands, nails, and cuticles before meeting others. Men should have short, well groomed nails. Women's nails should be "reasonably" long (that is, they don't get in the way as you go about daily activities). If you wear nail polish, manicure your nails the night before your presentation. Chipped nails are more noticeable than you might think.

REPEATED HAND MANNERISMS

Watch what other people do with their hands as they speak either formally in a presentation or informally in conversation. Notice repeated habits of touching the face, brushing hair back, scratching any one spot repeatedly, and other annoying, unnecessary movements. Some people choose to tap their fingers, click a pen, or shuffle papers just to have something to do with their hands. Become aware of your own hands and practice keeping them still except to gesture.

GENERAL BAD MANNERS

This category can encompass everything from looking everywhere except at the person you're talking with to interrupting others without listening to what they have to say. If you have a habit of consistently arriving late, using crude language, or rubbing your ear, improve those habits before your presentation. Be especially conscious of using time well. It is rude and inconsiderate to take more time for your presentation than you have been allotted. Begin and end on time. Because we are often the last to know of our own bad habits, try to think of times that friends or family have subtly suggested you improve something about yourself or gently teased you about one of your traits. Usually these people want to help you.

Remember that we only have one chance to make a positive first impression. That impression can last a lifetime. We may not be able to control our genetic makeup, our body type, height or facial features, but we can control the way we dress, wear our hair, and our general grooming habits. We also control our manners and demeanor.

When giving a presentation, even the best use of non-verbal skills can't make bad content good, but it can certainly affect how the audience receives good content. Using excellent nonverbal skills can improve your presentation measurably.

Learn more about nonverbal communication in the following exercises.

Exercises

NONWORDS

Objective

To become aware of your chronic patterns of using non-words (um, ah, like, you know, etc.).

Tools

The tools for this exercise include pingpong balls, wadded-up paper, or spud guns. (Spud guns are available in many toy stores. They are small, plastic, air-powered guns that shoot small potato pellets. The guns are not powerful enough for anyone to get hurt!)

Method

Note: This exercise should be used in a group setting with a friendly, very supportive atmosphere only. Trust within the group must be high.

A speaker with habitual use of nonwords must give his permission before a group uses this exercise. Before the presentation begins, each member of the audience is armed with tools (balls, papers, or guns). As the speaker begins, the audience listens attentively. Any time the speaker performs the agreed-on negative habit (ums, you-knows, etc.), a few members shoot their weapons at the speaker. The audience continues to shoot every time they hear or see the negative behavior.

Even though this seems like a ridiculous exercise, it is an excellent and positive way to eliminate bad habits.

This experience usually elicits lots of laughs and really makes the speaker aware of annoying habits. The next time the group meets, each speaker should repeat this exercise to note just how much he or she has improved! When everyone agrees to make this fun and not embarrassing, it really works!

THE "UM" GAME

Objective

To become aware of times when we use nonwords.

Method

In a classroom setting or with any group that would like to improve presentation skills, try this game for catching "filler" words. Form triads (groups of three) and assign roles. Each participant acts as either Speaker 1, Speaker 2, or Observer. Speakers 1 and 2 are asked to begin a conversation about any topic. The observer sets a timer and gives the signal to "go." The observer then listens for the speakers to use filler words like these:

Um. . .
Uh. . .
Ah. . .
Like. . .
You know. . .

The observer keeps score, giving one point to each player who uses one of the listed words. Scores are best kept with a hash mark system on a single sheet of paper. At the end of 3 minutes, the scores are totaled and the low score wins the competition. The group then changes roles until each person has served in all three roles. If several triads are competing, the low scorer from each triad can then compete with low scorers from other groups until a champion is found.

Repeat this game frequently. It is a humorous way to become aware of all the extraneous sounds we make. This kind of exercise, which makes us aware of the nonwords we use, is the *best* way to eliminate those annoying sounds.

UNPLANNED DANCING
Objective

To become aware of distracting foot movements or weight shifting.

Tools

The tools for this exercise include only a newspaper or sheets of paper from a flip chart.

Method

Place the paper on the floor beneath the speaker. Whenever the speaker moves his feet or shifts weight, the paper rustles and reminds him that he should move only when appropriate.

OBSERVATIONS

Objectives

To become conscious of specific effective and ineffective nonverbal cues.

To choose which nonverbal techniques are appropriate for you to use.

Method

Assume the role of a secret observer. Watch three speakers in different settings. Choose formal and informal settings, live or on film.

Watch for gestures, facial expressions, and body movements, focusing on one category at a time.

Take notes on the conscious or unconscious techniques each speaker uses.

Determine if the nonverbal cues are in synch with the verbal message.

Decide which gestures are effective for a formal speech but may not be for an informal setting. Remember that the same technique may be effective or ineffective depending on things like timing, overuse, intentionality, and setting.

Record your thoughts and observations on the grid on the next page.

Speaker Observations

Speaker _____ Occasion _____

	Effective	Ineffective	Why?
Technique 1			
Technique 2			
Technique 3			
Technique 4			

Things to Look For

Vocal techniques: Range, pitch, volume, articulation, rate, rhythm, pronunciation, nonwords, repetition, etc.

Body language: Gestures, appearance, eye contact, facial expressions, nervous hand or foot movements, pacing, etc.

TIME AWARENESS

Objective

To develop your "internal clock" so that you'll know when you've spoken for your assigned time limit whether it is 5, 10, or 30 minutes.

Method

Purchase or borrow a digital timer. They are available on digital watches, at kitchen stores, or even on your microwave! Set the time for your assigned limit and begin practicing your presentation without any breaks. Do not look at the timer during your first few practices. After you have developed an internal sense of how long it takes to get from start to finish of the speech, you may want to time each segment individually.

Chapter 15

Persuading an Audience

A student gave a powerful presentation on raising the national speed limit from 55 mph to 65 mph. At the conclusion of the presentation, he asked for a show of hands to indicate how many wanted to raise the speed limit. The entire class of 30 students responded affirmatively. Then he went on to ask how many would sign a prewritten letter addressed to the appropriate congressperson urging the law change.

Only 10 people raised their hands. When he went on to ask how many would mail the letter, only three students volunteered to take action. So even though the audience members were persuaded and sympathetic, they still wouldn't act.

Persuasion is difficult. Even when the audience feels you're right, they won't always act.

Five Steps to Persuasion

To persuade an audience, practice the following five steps:

1. Gain the audience's attention with a benefit or at least establish mutual goals or common ground.
2. Define the problem that will be solved if the request is approved.
3. Explain the solutions showing how the advantages of the solutions outweigh any negatives.
4. Enumerate the benefits to the audience.
5. State the specific action you want the audience to take.

Example

You need to gain support for an AIDS walk in a downtown area. You must speak to a group of retired people. Historically, this group isn't passionate about AIDS because they view it as a "younger person's disease" and as the product of an immoral society. How can you apply the five steps of persuasion?

1. You might start with statistics on older people who contracted AIDS from blood transfusions. Make the information familiar to the audience. Refer to sources or experts they respect, such as a well-known surgeon general or official of the AARP. This gives them reason to listen to you.

2. Then describe the problem of AIDS and whom it now affects. This might include their children and even grandchildren.

3. Describe how participating financially or physically in the walk helps solve the AIDS problem. Dispel any constraints or reasons for not participating.

4. Give the benefits the audience will receive from participating. Don't forget to list tangible and nontangible benefits. (A tangible result is the money raised from the walk. Nontangible results include helping the potential victims like grandchildren or their friends, and the good feeling that comes from volunteering.)

5. Ask them to sign up *now* either to sponsor a walker or to walk themselves. Without this action step, you may persuade them and leave with no result!

Persuasion Checklist

Many persuasive techniques apply to both speaking and writing. An excellent list of ten basic rules that can help you persuade an audience comes from *Power-Packed Writing That Works*, published by Communication Briefings, Alexandria, VA, 1989. Apply the following list to your next persuasive speech.

1. Know your audience.
2. Know what you can accomplish.
3. Anticipate objections.
4. Stress rewards.
5. Be familiar.

6. Be clear.
7. Ask for what you want.
8. Control the tone.
9. Clinch you argument.
10. Give them something to remember.

KNOW YOUR AUDIENCE.

Because the audience determines the effectiveness of your messages, you should conduct a standard audience analysis to determine demographics, attitudes, and values. However, effective persuasion requires you to consider one more audience characteristic: Is your audience active or passive? An *active audience* seeks out information and may already want to hear your presentation. *Passive audiences* aren't even thinking about you or your presentation.

According to James Grunig, researcher and professor at University of Maryland, stress *features* to active audiences and *benefits* to passive audiences. Cater to the agenda of an active audience by picturing the payoff for active audiences. Emphasize results.

Give passive audiences a problem. To gain attention quickly, find a problem that matters to them. Remember that adults learn best from examples. Quote others and provide examples from individuals your audience respects. Use memorable phrases like slogans, to reinforce your message. If you can determine the audience's agenda—what they want—you may persuade them.

KNOW WHAT YOU CAN ACCOMPLISH.

Don't expect to change the world with one speech. If you can move audience members from extremely negative to somewhat negative, you have succeeded. Set reasonable goals.

ANTICIPATE AND DISPEL OBJECTIONS.

Many audiences have significant reasons for not doing what you ask. These are their constraints or objections.

Example

You may persuade your audience to take a cruise to Cabo San Lucas. Though they are ready to pack their bags, they have no money. That's a constraint!

If you know the audience's constraints, you can dispel them one by one. With few constraints, the audience becomes available for persuasion.

Example

If you speak on the topic of abortion to a group of clergy who teach at a Catholic college, anticipate objections. Some of your audience will probably object to your topic. Dispel their objections by appealing to their role as educators. Note the number of college age women who choose abortion and stress the audience's need to know about and understand the procedure in order to deal with the students

STRESS REWARDS.

Point out the benefits of your proposal. Help the audience envision what will happen to them. Let them *see* and feel the difference. When you stress the benefits they receive from your suggestion, you keep the attention of both positive and negative audiences.

BE FAMILIAR.

When the audience can relate to the speaker, the chance of persuading them is greater.

Examples

To convince high school students not to drink and drive, a young victim of a drunk driving accident is a more effective speaker than a police officer.

You should not send a young person to persuade senior citizens to vote for an increased school budget.

The audience sees a familiar person as credible.

BE CLEAR.

If the audience has to make a great effort to understand, they won't act. Develop your argument simply and make your request clear and uncomplicated.

ASK FOR WHAT YOU WANT.

Sometimes a speaker develops a powerful argument for the audience to act, then forgets to tell them what happens next. Don't underestimate the value of simply saying what you want the audience to do. Make their job easy. Remember the speed limit example? The speaker asked the audience to act by sending a letter to a congressperson. If he hadn't asked, even the three people wouldn't have acted for him.

CONTROL THE TONE.

Establish a relationship with the audience by the words you use. The *first person*, or "I," signifies authority. This might work if you are an expert. Otherwise it could annoy the audience because they don't identify with you. The *second person*, or "you," signifies familiarity. The "I" attitude focuses on the speaker and excludes the audience. The "you" attitude includes the audience and sounds conversational. Use the *third person*, "he, she, it, the company," when you want to signify objectivity. Sometimes objectivity works well in persuasion, particularly if you don't want to appear personally involved when presenting facts or supporting materials.

CLINCH YOUR ARGUMENT.

Use a powerful reason that the audience and speaker both accept. Commonly held beliefs and attitudes are clinchers. If your audience agrees with your clincher, they probably agree with your overall proposal.

Example

Purpose: We, the school board, need to enlarge our middle school so that our children can receive instruction in an appropriate setting.

Evidence: Several hundred students now crowd in trailers for classrooms.

Clincher: You'll agree that the personal attention and quality instruction we seek for our children cannot happen in these crowded, nonconducive trailers.

GIVE THEM SOMETHING TO REMEMBER.

Use a brief memorable phrase that sums up what you said. A motto or unique phrase helps retention.

Examples

Most of us know what Smokey the Bear says: "Only you can prevent forest fires."

Nike is known for "Just do it."

If your audience remembers the message, you may change opinions. Provide a handout or something they can take with them if they decide to act later.

Try the following exercises to practice persuasive techniques.

Exercise

USING PERSUASIVE ELEMENTS

Objective

To identify persuasive elements.

Method

Read the following presentation and identify all the persuasive elements listed in this chapter.

To Use or Not to Use: Belts or Bags

I never used to wear a seatbelt, having heard horror stories about Jessica Savich, a news anchor, imprisoned in her car as she drowned in two feet of water. I had heard stories of cars that burst into flames when hit from behind. Surely a seatbelt would make it too hard to get out of these situations.

Then, one fall day as I drove quickly along to work, my car slid on wet leaves. I hit the driver's side of an older gentleman's car. When I looked down to see if I was intact, everything looked fine. Then, I looked in the mirror. My teeth looked like Dracula. The top four teeth distended much lower than normal. All that orthodontic work for nothing! The next thing I knew, the ambulance arrived to take me and the man I hit to the emergency room

When my accident happened, few cars had airbags. Today, most cars have them. Should we still wear seatbelts? The National Traffic Safety Control Board indicates that almost 85% of the public now uses seatbelts even though their cars also contain airbags. Research indicates that in over 90% of accidents, seatbelts help rather than hinder you. For the two horror stories I told you earlier, hundreds of thousands of stories feature fatalities because no seatbelt was worn.

Many of us young businesspeople feel invincible, just as I did until I hit that car. Then I started wearing a seatbelt religiously, airbag or no airbag. You're probably aware that most airbags only cushion your accident if you're hit head on. Since that accident, I have been hit twice. Once I was broadsided and no airbag emerged; the other time, I was hit on the right rear side and again, no airbag emerged. Because I wore a seatbelt, both times I walked away injury-free. The damage to the vehicle was significant—almost $10,000 the first time and $5,000 the second.

You can save a valuable life—your own. And you won't have to worry about hitting a scared older gentleman and ruining his car. The dental specialist who operated on me said that I hit my four teeth squarely on the steering wheel. If I had worn a seatbelt, I could have avoided the operation. Wear your seatbelt religiously— even if you have four airbags. Your family and friends will be glad you did.

To Use or Not to Use: Belts or Bags

(Gain attention.) I never used to wear a seatbelt, having heard horror stories about Jessica Savich, a news anchor, imprisoned in her car as she drowned in two feet of water. I had heard stories of cars that burst into flames when hit from behind. **(Anticipate objections.)** Surely a seatbelt would make it too hard to get out of these situations.

Then, one fall day as I drove quickly along to work, my car slid on wet leaves. I hit the driver's side of an older gentleman's car. When I looked down to see if I was intact, everything looked fine. Then, I looked in the mirror. My teeth looked like Dracula. The top four teeth distended much lower than normal. All that orthodontic work for nothing! The next thing I knew, the ambulance arrived to take me and the man I hit to the emergency room

(Define problem.) When my accident happened, few cars had airbags. Today, most cars have them. Should we still wear seatbelts? The National Traffic Safety Control Board indicates that almost 85% of the public now uses seatbelts even though their cars also contain airbags. **(Dispel objections.)** Research indicates that in over 90% of accidents, seatbelts help rather than hinder you. For the two horror stories I told you earlier, hundreds of thousands of stories feature fatalities because no seatbelt was worn.

(Be familiar.) Many of us young businesspeople feel invincible, just as I did until I hit that car. **(Control the tone.)** Then, I started wearing a seatbelt religiously, airbag or no airbag. You're probably aware that most airbags only cushion your accident if you're hit head on. Since that accident, I have been hit twice. Once I was broadsided and no airbag emerged; the other time, I was hit on the right rear side and again, no airbag emerged. **(Evidence.)** Because I wore a seatbelt, both times I walked away injury-free. The damage to the vehicle was significant—almost $10,000 the first time and $5,000 the second.

(Benefit.) You can save a valuable life—your own. **(Benefit.)** And you won't have to worry about hitting a scared older gentleman and ruining his car. The dental specialist who operated on me said that I hit my four teeth squarely on the steering wheel. If I had worn a seatbelt, I could have avoided the operation. **(Action.)** Wear your seatbelt religiously—even if you have four airbags. **(Clincher.)** Your family and friends will be glad you did.

TOY BAG GAME

Objectives

To practice using persuasive techniques.

To develop appropriate persuasive approaches for different audiences.

Method

This exercise works well in a group setting but can be done individually with the assistance of a video camera. The group leader brings a canvas bag of assorted odd items. A sample bag might contain these things:

- Slinky
- Clay
- Tape measure
- Play money
- Badminton shuttlecock
- Sunglasses

The participants reach into the bag and draw out an item without looking. Each speaker has 4 minutes to develop a 1-minute "sales pitch" for their item. Use the persuasive techniques listed in the chapter. Envision different audiences. Develop different persuasive techniques for two audiences. The intended use for each item *cannot* be used; however, new uses, statistics, and history can be fabricated. Present your sales pitch and review your videotape to check how well you performed.

Chapter 16

Are There Any Questions?

Many presentations include a question-and-answer period. The time when questions are asked can affect the tone of your speech. It's important to be honest, in control, and confident. Before you speak, determine when and how you'll take questions.

When to Take Questions

QUESTIONS WITHIN A PRESENTATION

The advantage to taking questions throughout your presentation is that any confusion your listeners have can be clarified immediately and you can speak directly to their concerns. The major disadvantage is that the sequence, emphasis, and your major message can get lost when you give "floor time" to audience members. Any listener with his own agenda can "grandstand" during your allotted time. But taking questions during your performance tends to give the presentation a more informal tone and may be the best technique to use with small groups of under 25. Questions offered during a talk require flexibility and often demand more time for the total presentation.

QUESTIONS AFTER THE PRESENTATION

Holding questions until the end of your speech allows you to maintain control. You have the opportunity to make important points at the time you choose to make them. The disadvantage is that you may have overlooked sharing some information and some of the audience may be lost. A simple clarification in response to a question might have eliminated some confusion.

Techniques for Fielding Questions

- *Answer the question being asked.* Sometimes speakers look foolish when they answer the question they anticipated rather than the question really posed. Listen carefully to the question before formulating your answer.

- *Repeat the question so that the entire audience can hear.* Answer each part of compound questions separately.

- *Rephrase any complicated, hostile, or confusing questions.* Use a neutral tone to rephrase any leading or biased questions. If a questioner remains openly hostile toward your topic, offer to speak with him after the presentation

- *If you don't know an answer, don't fake it.* When you fake an answer, you risk losing credibility with the listeners. An honest response is the best approach. If you're asked a question that you can't answer, you can refer the question to an audience member who has more expertise or promise to find the answer and get back to the questioner.

- *Think of each answer as a tiny speech.* When answering a question you feel was not covered completely, use an introduction, main points, and a conclusion.

- *Look directly at the questioner as you begin your answer.* As you continue with your answer, include the entire audience with your eye contact. Conclude your answer by looking back at the questioner. If the questioner dominates the Q&A period, do not look back at him as you conclude your answer. Turn your eyes to another part of the room and ask for more questions.

- *If you are limited by time or if the questioner is dominating your time, avoid asking, "Did I answer your question?"* If you are teaching, complete understanding is critical, "Did I answer your question?" may be an appropriate response.

- *Rephrase your answer if asked a question you have previously answered.* Attempt to help the questioner save face and not be embarrassed for repeating a question.

Example

If a questioner asks how you reached your conclusion, you might respond this way: "We reached our conclusion by working through the four steps I mentioned. Then we drew final conclusions based on the results in step four."

This is a straight, simple response that should not make the questioner feel stupid. Avoid saying "As I *just* said. . . ."

- *If asked a question you will cover soon, give a brief answer and promise a more thorough explanation in a few moments.*

Example

If you are explaining a process and a questioner asks for the bottom line, you might answer: "The bottom line is seventy-five thousand dollars and in just a moment I'd like to explain how I reached that figure. First, I think it's important to quickly conclude my explanation of the process we used."

- *Answer as concisely as possible.* Don't get sidetracked or ramble.

- *As you prepare your presentation, anticipate likely questions.* Come prepared with statistics and examples to support your responses.

- *If no one asks a question on a point you would like to reiterate, you have at least two options:* You can "plant" someone in the audience to ask the essential question or ask the question yourself. You might say, "Some of you may be wondering . . ." and then follow with the information you want to give.

- *If the audience is hesitant to ask questions, encourage them by asking each one to find a partner and discuss any questions he/she might have.* After two or three minutes ask what questions were unanswered. This normally helps a shy audience to speak out.

- *When the question-and-answer period has ended, give a brief wrap-up and restate your conclusion.* If you ask the audience to do something, now is the time to repeat your request.

Remember that you have the most power with an audience at the beginning and end of a presentation.

Practice ways to handle question with the following exercises.

Exercises

PRACTICING ANSWERS

Objective

To become more comfortable answering questions before a group.

Method

Ask a friend to help you or use this method or practice with a group. A number of books on the market consist of questions for which there are no right answers, such as *If*, Volumes 1, 2, and 3, *The Book of Questions*, and many others.

Practice answering questions you've chosen at random (without thinking about them in advance). Phrase your answers in the format you will want to use for your presentation. If you are practicing for an impromptu presentation, try answering in the format of introduction, body (with three main points), and a conclusion that ties back to the introduction. Take 1 minute to think before you answer, and speak for 2 minutes. Ask your listeners to tell you when 2 minutes have elapsed.

Video tape yourself during this exercise. Sometimes we behave differently in an impromptu setting and you'll want to see how well you perform!

Chapter 17

Group Presentations

Most of the basic rules that apply to a single-speaker presentation apply to group presentations. Group presentations are often used for work group or project team reports, major sales meetings, and panels. The purposes of featuring a team of speakers are to:

- Showcase the knowledge of team members.
- Introduce key members of the hierarchy.
- Keep variety in a long presentation.

Some organizations may have politically oriented reasons for choosing a team format. This occurs when the key members of the work team are poor presenters.

Many organizations pay speech consultants thousands of dollars to improve their group presentation style, especially for sales or marketing presentations. These companies know that they are simply investing in their future. Successful presentations can result in millions of dollars in sales and thousands of dollars worth of goodwill. The cost of poor presentations is hard to measure because we don't know "what might have been." Here are some tips for preparing and presenting presentations involving more than one speaker.

Preparing for Group Presentations

- *Use preparation time wisely.* Make clear assignments to avoid time lost due to confusion. Arrive for meetings on time. Use e-mail when possible.

- *Practice the presentation together once to emphasize content, checking for consistent terms.* Practice several more times to assure that transitions from speaker to speaker are seamless. Your words as well as your physical movements should appear smooth, natural, and professional.

- *Each person involved should be prepared to "fill in" in case one presenter is sick or unable to do her part.*

- *Not every member of a large group has to speak during the presentation.* Four to six presenters is an ideal number. Fewer than four speakers may not seem representative of the group, and the transitions between more than six speakers may appear choppy. Other participants can be assigned to gather data, make the visual aids, or prepare the script and notes. Everyone representing the group should be available to answer questions.

- *Prepare visual aids that use consistent fonts, colors, and styles.* When possible, one person should prepare visual aids for the entire team. This ensures a consistent appearance.

- *Know the exact physical setup before the group arrives.* Prepare and practice using that setup. If the room is rearranged when you arrive, return it to the agreed-on style if possible. If you can't change the arrangement, hold a quick discussion among group members to determine any adjustments you must make.

- *Panel members should dress in a consistent style.* A mix of suits and jeans sends a mixed message to the audience. Dress to match the setting, the topic and the expectations of the audience. (Students shouldn't wear torn jeans or T-shirts with questionable sayings!)

Presenting in a Group

- *Listen carefully to each other speak.* Pay special attention during the question-and-answer period. Don't "step on each other's lines," which means don't begin speaking until other panel members have finished. If a question has been answered incompletely or needs to be clarified, other panel members should feel free to add to the answer. Do so tactfully and without making the first speaker or group feel embarrassed.

- *While one person from the group is speaking, all other members should keep their eyes on the presenter.* Remember that the whole panel is "on stage" before, during, and after the presentation. Give full attention to the speaker— don't look around the room, practice your speech, or talk with someone else on your panel.

- *Observe the agreed-on time limits for each segment.* Agree on a signal that the group members can use to indicate a speaker's time is up. The signal should be unrecognizable to the audience but clear to the group.

- *When the formal part of the presentation ends, the body posture of all members should be consistent.* All should sit or stand to take questions. The last speaker should not be the only one "left standing" because audience members are then tempted to direct all questions to that person.

- *At the end of the question-and-answer period, one person must be prepared to give a quick wrapup, reviewing the most important points.*

For any group presentation, think *team*. Work together, support each other, and emphasize the best skills of each speaker.

Exercise

MAKING THEM WORK

Objective

To prepare for group presentations.

Method

Review the following situations and answer the questions for each. Keep in mind the techniques you have learned in previous chapters.

Situation 1

Four students are required to give a presentation to the board of trustees at their university. The subject is the need for a new health center.

1. How should they dress for the presentation? _____

   _____

   _____

2. How should they gather information for their presentation? _____

   _____

   _____

3. How should they check the accuracy of that information? _____

   _____

   _____

4. What visual aids should they use?_____

   _____

   _____

5. How should the materials be prepared and how should the students practice using them?_____

   _____

   _____

Situation 2

   The entire executive management team of an engineering company as well as a project manager and several key team members have been selected as finalists for a major work project. Two other companies are also under consideration. Receiving the contract for this project could result in millions of dollars for the company. There are 15 members of the selected team and five audience members present for the final presentation.

1. The team will present in the company conference room and arrange the chairs and tables any way it wants. What arrangement would you suggest the team choose? ____

   _____

   _____

2. What type of presentation is this—informative or persuasive? _____

_____

_____

3. How many team members should speak? _____

_____

_____

Part IV

Postcript:
Do's and Don'ts

Chapter 1: Getting Started

Do

- Immediately brainstorm a list of possible ideas for your presentation.
- Determine your purpose statement.
- Keep your specific statement in mind at all times.
- Keep a positive attitude.
- Choose a training environment to interact with your audience.
- Use notes for public speaking.
- Know the difference between public speaking and training.

Don't

- Feel you are limited only to items on your idea list.
- Speak for more than one hour.
- Speak when you should train.
- Procrastinate or panic!

Chapter 2: Fear Fighting

Do

- Think of yourself as an Olympian in training.
- Start your preparation early.
- Practice with a video camera.
- Practice in a room similar to the one in which you will actually speak.
- Exercise briefly before your presentation to eliminate excess adrenaline.

Don't

- Eat a hearty meal, consume large quantities of caffeine, milk, or sugar.
- Hesitate to ask a coach to give you feedback.
- Focus on your fear.

Chapter 3: Getting Acquainted with Your Audience

Do

- Know the demographics of the audience before you prepare your presentation.
- Choose language appropriate to the knowledge level of the audience.
- Choose topics that interest your audience.
- Speak to the concerns of the audience.
- Know why they are gathered.

Don't

- Use acronyms extensively.
- Use sexist, racist, or offensive language.
- Use inappropriate examples.
- Make sweeping assumptions about the group.

Chapter 4: Gathering Data

Do

- Use multiple sources to find data—library, internet, interviews, material from organizations, personal experiences, etc.
- Use statistics and facts to back up your statements.
- Send a thank-you note following an interview.
- Familiarize yourself with the Internet.
- Use only credible Internet sources.

Don't

- Forget to double check your information.
- Wait to schedule an interview—most people need as much advance notice as possible.
- Expect a librarian to do your research for you.

Chapter 5: Presenting Data

Do

- State a statistic, then rephrase it in easily comprehensible terms.
- Support numbers with pictures when possible.
- Use a pie chart to show percentages.
- Use a bar graph or line graph to compare data over time.
- When possible, use color to emphasize differences.

Don't

- Make graphs too complicated.
- Neglect to label each axis of charts and graphs.
- Use a graph that doesn't clearly distinguish between pieces of data.
- Read a string of numbers.

Chapter 6: Organizing Your Information

Do

- Use a chronological pattern when you tell a story.
- Use a logical, spatial pattern when your topic can be divided by location.
- Choose a topical pattern when information is best divided into categories.
- Use a causal pattern when one thing occurs as a direct result of another.
- Use a problem-solution pattern when your goal is to convince the audience that one solution is superior to all others.

Don't

- Include information that does not fit into your selected pattern.
- Mix organizational patterns within a speech.
- Prepare your presentation randomly without using an organizational pattern.

Chapter 7: Introductions

Do

- Get the audience involved.
- Create interest in the topic of your presentation.
- Speak clearly and with confidence.
- Establish common ground with the audience.
- Get the attention of the audience.
- Let the audience know "What's in it for them?"
- Choose an introductory technique that is appropriate for your topic.

Don't

- Start any presentation with "I'm gonna tell you about . . . ."
- Use a long-winded introduction.
- Use a false start like, "Before I begin, I want to tell you . . . ."
- Use a canned joke.
- Name drop to impress.
- Start speaking before you've reached the lectern.
- Let your introduction sound memorized.
- Apologize for anything—nervousness, forgetting hand-outs, or spilling coffee on your shirt.
- Use an overly emotional introduction. Sad, sentimental, bittersweet and touching are okay; gut-wrenching is not.
- Start speaking before your props, notes, and equipment are in place.
- Make a presumptive statement like, "Everybody loves baseball" or "I'm sure you all plan to get married some day."
- Ask a question that they may perceive as silly and could turn off your audience like, "Did you ever wonder why cows eat grass?"
- Spend a lot of time in your introduction building a relationship if the audience already knows you.

Chapter 8: Conclusions

Do

- Conclude with emphasis.
- Call the audience to action if your goal is to persuade.
- Remind the audience why your topic is important to them.
- Refer to the introduction when appropriate.
- Answer a question you asked in your introduction.

Don't

- Say ". . . and I guess that's about it."
- Say "and in conclusion . . ." and then go on to another topic.
- Apologize for taking their time, getting lost in your notes, your shaking hands, the temperature of the room, etc.
- Mumble your last sentence.
- Add, "Oh, one more thing . . ." to the end of your conclusion.
- Gather up your notes and props while you're still speaking.
- Let your voice trail off and not finish your last sentence.
- Forget to practice your conclusion.

Chapter 9: Outlining

Do

- Follow standard outline procedures.
- Match every A with a B.
- Use complete sentences.
- Write out the introduction and conclusion.
- Include transitional phrases.

Don't

- List multiple points within one symbol.

- Use more than five points.
- Leave out any sections of the speech.

Chapter 10: Physical Environment

Do

- Use theater style for large groups.
- Use "U" style for maximum interaction with the audience.
- Avoid long, narrow rooms.
- Keep the room cool.
- Allow for desks or tables when training.

Don't

- Choose a room too large or too small for the audience size.
- Allow outside noises to distract your audience.
- Use only lighting from above.

Chapter 11: Using Notes That Work for You

Do

- Number your note cards.
- Print with large, legible letters.
- Use white paper.
- Keep a second copy of your notes in a separate place from your original copy.
- Use colors for different sections of your notes.
- Write out quotes and statistics.
- Rehearse using your actual notes.
- Include stage directions for yourself.
- Use a minimum size of 18-point type.
- Use as few cards as possible.

Don't

- Write in full sentences.
- Write on both sides of the cards.
- Hold note cards rather than place them on a lectern.
- Look at the cards except when you really need to read them.
- Memorize your speech verbatim rather than using the cards.

Chapter 12: Visual Aids

Do

- Supplement words with visual aids.
- Prepare visuals in advance.
- Keep it simple.
- Use large print.
- Use meaningful visual aids.
- Use color for accent.
- Time the way you use visuals.
- Keep extra copies of all visuals.
- Explain any visual you use.

Don't

- Use slides when the audience needs to see the speaker's face.
- Put too many words on a visual.
- Talk to a prop or visual.
- Panic if your computer fails.
- Block the view of a slide or transparency.
- Pass items around the room if they will distract from your words.
- *Read!*

Chapter 13: Keeping Them Tuned In

Do

- Use your natural voice.
- Use a wide vocal range.
- Project from the diaphragm.
- Use dictionary pronunciation.
- Use words that create a picture for the listener.
- Repeat for retention.
- Use ear-friendly words.

Don't

- Speak too softly.
- Race to the end.
- Slur your words.
- Use complicated words or phrases.
- Use regional terminology.

Chapter 14: What You Don't Say Speaks Louder than Words

Do

- Keep appropriate eye contact.
- Plant your feet a shoulder width apart.
- Shake hands firmly.
- Use good manners.

Don't

- Stand motionless or pace.
- Slouch.
- Say "um," "ah," "like," or "you know" as fillers.
- Unconsciously repeat certain phrases.
- Wear sloppy clothes.

Chapter 15: Persuading an Audience

Do

- Dress, act, and speak in a way that is familiar to your audience.
- Establish common ground with an audience.
- Anticipate and dispel objections.
- Use the appropriate tone (I, you, he, she, etc.).
- Ask an audience to act immediately for you.
- Give them something to remember.

Don't

- Assume the audience is sympathetic and will take action.
- Forget to provide options or choices for your audience.
- Allow the audience to leave without acting.
- Try to accomplish too much in one presentation.
- Use unclear messages or language.
- Fail to clinch your argument.

Chapter 16: Are There Any Questions

Do

- Anticipate and prepare for questions.
- Rephrase biased or leading questions.
- Use an introduction, body, and conclusion in your answer.
- Repeat questions so that all can hear.
- Let the audience know if you'll take questions during or after the presentation.

Don't

- Ask "Did I answer your question?" if pressed for time or if the questioner dominates the Q&A period.

- Get sidetracked or ramble during an answer.
- Rush to answer before you have heard the whole question.

Chapter 17: Group Presentations

Do

- Practice the presentation together as a group.
- Have an understudy for each speaker.
- Practice transitions between speakers.
- Choose the best physical arrangement for the room.
- Use consistent fonts and colors for each visual aid.
- Dress consistently and appropriately.
- Listen intently as other group members speak.

Don't

- Ask more than six group members to speak.
- Hesitate to add more information to an answer offered by another group member.
- Ignore time limits.
- Leave one member standing at the end of the presentation.
- Forget to add a powerful conclusion after the question-and-answer period.

Index